KEEPING UP THE GOOD WORK

A Practitioner's Guide to Mental Health Ethics

Fourth Edition

Leonard J. Haas, PhD
and
John L. Malouf, PhD

Professional Resource Press
Sarasota, Florida

Published by Professional Resource Press
(An imprint of Professional Resource Exchange, Inc.)
Post Office Box 15560
Sarasota, FL 34277-1560

This publication is sold with the understanding that the Publisher is not engaged in rendering professional services. If legal, psychological, medical, accounting, or other expert advice or assistance is sought or required, the reader should seek the services of a competent professional.

The copy editor for this book was David Anson, the typesetter was Denise Franck, the managing editor was Debbie Fink, the production coordinator was Laurie Girsch, and Carol Tornatore created the cover.

Library of Congress Cataloging-in-Publication Data

Haas, Leonard J.
  Keeping up the good work : a practitioner's guide to mental
health ethics / Leonard J. Haas and John L. Malouf.--4th ed.
    p. ; cm.
  Includes bibliographical references and index.
  ISBN 1-56887-092-2 (alk. paper)
    1. Mental health personnel--Professional ethics. 2. Psychiatric
ethics. I. Malouf, John L. II. Title.

RC455.2.E8 H33 2005
174'.2--dc22
                                            2004060089

TABLE OF CONTENTS

PREFACE

Although mental health practice has never been simple or stress free, it seems to many of us that the strains are increasing and that the role of mental health practitioners is becoming more complicated. Practitioners are continually faced with the pressures of economic survival, such as receiving third-party reimbursement, collecting from clients, and justifying the necessity for mental health services to utilization reviewers. Additionally, the watershed *Tarasoff* decision began a trend to enlarge clinicians' responsibilities for the potential actions of their patients that has continued and shows no sign of abating.

When confronted by this multiplicity of demands and obligations, practitioners unfortunately may neglect to pay adequate attention to the ethical standards and values that should guide their practice. Instead, we may compromise or confuse such standards in the face of more immediate practical, financial, or legal considerations. The practice of giving a patient a diagnosis because it is reimbursable by insurance companies; accepting an individual as a patient, even though one has no demonstrable competence in treating the problem presented; and "ethics" workshops that are in reality aimed at avoiding lawsuits are all examples of situations in which ethical considerations are sacrificed for the sake of other requirements. Even in the best of circumstances, the ethical course of action is often not easy or clear-cut.

Our motivation for writing this book was to aid clinical practitioners in understanding and applying ethical principles in their practices. The various topics we cover represent those areas of professional practice where ethical concerns are dominant or where practitioners commonly misunderstand their ethical obligations or options.

We are aware that much of what has been written concerning professional ethics has been so general and theoretical that it is difficult for practitioners to apply the information in their practices. In response to this limitation, we have attempted to apply solid ethical principles to the practical problems professionals face daily. Although many if not most ethical problems defy hard and fast rules, several chapters in this book present relevant questions or guidelines that practitioners should consider in making a decision. The guidelines presented should focus the reader's attention on relevant issues and aid in decision making. Some of what we have written may seem to simply represent common knowledge or good judgment. Nonetheless, much "common knowledge" is overlooked in the course of a busy practice. We hope that, by reading and thinking about these issues, practitioners will be more deliberate in their practical decisions. We have also tried to maintain a helpful and positive attitude. Such an orientation reflects our belief that the vast majority of mental health professionals sincerely want to provide ethical services, but they also want to make a reasonable living and avoid getting sued.

This is not a book on legalities, although appropriate legal considerations will be considered in the light of the ethical issue being discussed. This is not a book on professionalism, although there are numerous occasions when making ethical decisions will bear upon aspects of professionalism. Nor is this a book on clinical strategies, although making ethical decisions clearly has a substantial effect on practitioners' clinical strategies. Rather, this *is* a book on clinical decisions of various sorts; we hope that readers will come to consider not only what is legally, practically, and clinically justified, but also what is ethical. Thus, we hope that through reading this book, practitioners will integrate higher levels of ethical behavior into their practices.

Further, this is not a book written solely for psychologists, despite the fact that both of the authors are psychologists. Rather, it *is* a book addressed to all clinical practitioners in the mental health professions. Although there are certain distinct differences in training, expertise, and prerogatives among the various professions, there are many more similarities than differences. All of the mental health disciplines share a sense of professionalism, a duty to provide for the welfare of clients or patients, and a commitment to improving standards of practice, among other things. We hope that this book will be useful both in graduate coursework and in professional development, to social workers, psychiatrists, marriage and family therapists, professional counselors, and other mental health workers in addition to psychologists.

Throughout this and the previous three editions, our attempt has been to raise issues of ethics and professional standards in a practical context and with respect for the realities of clinical practice. Although some chapters have stood the test of time since the first edition of this book, many chapters have been substantially revised. We have included the most recent revisions of the ethical codes of all the major mental health professions, and we have discussed their implications for practice. With this edition, we include the ethics code of the American Counseling Association, in addition to the revised codes of psychology, psychiatry, social work, and marriage and family therapy.

Like the professions' codes of ethics themselves, we have based this book on fundamental principles of professional ethics and then applied them to emerging developments in the mental health practice environment. In previous editions, we have expanded our focus to include the rise of new health care reimbursement schemes, the Internet, the increased use of preferred practice guidelines, empirically validated treatments, practice in forensic contexts, and electronic aspects of practice. In the current edition we have further expanded our consideration of the most recent dramatic change in the practice environment, the passage of the Health Insurance Portability and Accountability Act (HIPAA), which affects both privacy practices and record keeping.

There is little doubt that the importance of mental health services in society will continue to grow, and the contribution that practitioners can make will be increasingly significant. It is also our hope, and the purpose of this book, that our ethical behavior will keep up with these changes and continue to do honor to the mental health professions.

KEEPING UP THE GOOD WORK

A Practitioner's Guide to Mental Health Ethics

Fourth Edition

Chapter 1

THE NATURE OF PROFESSIONAL ETHICS

This chapter provides a brief discussion of the theory and philosophy underlying the practice of professional ethics. It deals with three questions: What is professional ethics? What makes an action ethical? Are there different types of ethical obligations?

WHAT IS ETHICS?

One useful method for distinguishing ethics from other major standards for determining whether an action is right, good, or proper is to contrast it with those frameworks. Law (especially criminal law) and etiquette can be thought of as domains similar to ethics because each focuses on aspects of proper or correct behavior, and each specifies penalties for deviation.

Even though each set of standards reflects in some respects the consensus of the society or culture which promotes it, moral frameworks are (or should be) developed largely through rational processes. Although obviously founded on moral concepts, legal standards in contrast are developed through political processes whereas norms of etiquette are developed for the most part by historical precedent and social utility.

Ethical standards, in theory at least, focus on behavior and on motivations that aim at the highest ideals of human behavior. Criminal law, in contrast, focuses primarily on proscribed behavior that may harm other members of the society, and etiquette focuses on behavior that establishes one's good standing within a subgroup.

1

Actions that violate moral or ethical standards can result in censure, guilt, or social criticism. Illegal behavior, on the other hand, results in actual punishment, if detected; impolite behavior results in social penalties—ostracism or perhaps mild social criticism.

In the view of many moral philosophers, ethics is distinguished by three main features: (a) it is based on *principles;* (b) the principles have *universality* (i.e., could be applied generally to all similar persons); and (c) appropriate behavior may be deduced from the principles by *reasoning.* Thus, ethics proper should involve adherence to a consistent set of principles assumed to be relevant for all individuals in similar situations, which result (deductively) in obligations to take particular actions.

Two relevant facts follow from this. First, codes of professional ethics are actually not pure ethics but rather a combination of ethics, law, and etiquette; and second, no existing ethical theory (especially no theory of professional ethics) meets the standard set forth above. Thus we are dealing with a somewhat indeterminate, evolving framework with which to guide decisions and actions. Despite this uncertainty, however, a code of professional ethics can indeed provide important guidance in developing one's model of good professional functioning.

THE NATURE OF PROFESSIONAL ETHICS

Although some may argue that professional ethics are distinct from general moral obligations (Beauchamp & Childress, 2001), it is clear that professionals (whether psychologists, psychiatrists, architects, lawyers, or marriage and family therapists) take on special duties to persons who enter professional relationships with them. Legally the special obligations of the professional are known as *fiduciary.* This term denotes the special duty to care for the welfare of those who have become one's clients or patients. The fact that the mental health practitioner is in a fiduciary relationship with clients implies to some writers that there are special ethical obligations. One example concerns loyalty; the psychotherapist cannot simply decide that he or she is no longer interested in treating a particular patient and discontinue treatment because this would constitute *abandonment.* This standard of loyalty is higher than that to which average citizens are held because they are free to terminate most voluntary relationships, such as friendships.

THE NATURE OF ETHICAL ACTS

As noted, actions are generally considered to be ethical if they have the following characteristics: First, they are *principled;* that is, the actor must be able to justify his or her actions in the light of some specific, generally accepted moral principles (e.g., honesty, duty to avoid harming others, respect for human dignity, preservation of freedom). Second, the action must be a *reasoned* outcome of consideration of the principles. This relates to the notion of free will in moral responsibility; that is, the actor is assumed to be capable of choice and thus responsible for basing his or her actions on ethical principles. Third, the action must be *universalizable;* that is, the actor must be able to recommend that others in similar situations do the same thing.

MAJOR TYPES OF ETHICAL JUSTIFICATIONS

Teleological Justification

Although the foregoing suggests that the inherent *features* of certain acts mark them as ethical, the question of their *consequences* can also be raised in this regard. The method of moral justification called *teleology* or *utilitarianism* indicates that an action is ethical if it results in the creation of more good than harm, or as Bentham (1863/1948) phrased it in his famous maxim, it produces "the greatest good for the greatest number." This principle has been criticized by ethical theorists because it may lead to "the ends justifying the means." Such criticisms of teleology frequently are based on *deontological* principles. Additional problems with teleological analyses focus on the problem of who is entitled to judge the "good" or "bad," which flows from a moral choice.

Deontological Justification

Deontology, a contrasting framework with which to justify the ethical quality of actions, posits that actions are ethical if they manifest one of a small set of primary moral characteristics. For example, in early versions of medical ethics, the preservation of life was the primary ethical principle. Thus, an action which was intended to preserve life was ethical regardless of what other consequences it produced. Using a deontological method of determining the rightness of one's actions becomes difficult when more than one moral principle is involved because deontology provides no decision rules for selecting the *more* ethical action when each choice is based on a different moral ground. For example, if telling the truth would result in someone's death (the famous example is that of the hospital administrator in Nazi-occupied Europe who is asked if there are any Jewish patients in the hospital), which is the proper course—to be honest or to preserve life? Criticisms of deontological methods of ethical justification focus on this problem (deontologically ethical actions creating evil results) as a demonstration of the inadequacy of the method.

VARIETIES OF ETHICAL OBLIGATIONS

Ethical obligations can be more or less explicit and can constitute either the minimally acceptable standard or the ideal to which the ethically responsible practitioner aspires. Minimal standards (the "floor" of ethics) are known as mandatory ethical obligations. Ideals (or the "ceiling" of ethics) are known as aspirational obligations (Gerts, 1981). Generally, one can be criticized or punished for violating mandatory obligations; additionally, one is typically not praised for successfully upholding them. Conversely, individuals are not commonly censured or punished for violating aspirational obligations; much more commonly, those who succeed in upholding such standards are commended and admired. In terms familiar to readers of the Ten Commandments, mandatory obligations can be thought of as "thou shalt not"s, while aspirational obligations can be thought of as "thou shalt"s. For example, the *Ethical Principles of Psychologists and Code of Conduct* (American Psychological Association, 2002) has as one of its mandatory ethical obligations the duty to refrain from "uninvited in-person solicitation of business" from potential clients. This injunction is based on the notion that the vulnerabilities of laypersons could be exploited by a mental health professional subtly or directly indicating the presence of a psychological problem. This can be seen as a "thou shalt not." It would be remarkable for a psychologist to be praised for avoiding such solicitation; on the other hand, it would be quite likely that such a practitioner would be censured for participating in such activities. Conversely, the principle embodied in the *Ethical Principles of Psychologists and Code of Conduct* to "respect the dignity and worth of all people" can be seen as an aspirational ethical obligation. It is difficult to determine when a professional has met this obligation, and it could easily be argued that the aim is never completely realized. Indeed, the conscientious practitioner devotes his or her entire professional career to achieving this end. Thus, it would be unusual for a practitioner to be censured for "failing to promote human dignity," while it would be much more common for a practitioner who exemplified exceptional ability to promote human dignity to be honored for this.

It is important not to confuse aspirational and mandatory obligations. If one believes that aspirational obligations are in fact mandatory (i.e., mistakes the ethical ceiling for the ethical floor), one runs the risk of feeling hopelessly inadequate as an ethical practitioner. This approach is not uncommonly seen among professionals in training when they are first exposed to education in professional ethics. They begin to believe that their obligations are so massive and overwhelming as to prevent them from ever functioning effectively as clinicians. Indeed, an important aspect of one's development as a competent, ethical mental health practitioner demands that one be continually aware of aspirational obligations, while at the same time avoiding the overwhelming sense of inadequacy that prevents experiencing any satisfaction with one's work.

Conversely, one can run the risk of confusing mandatory with aspirational obligations (i.e., mistaking the ethical floor for the ethical ceiling). In such cases the practitioner believes that even the explicitly stated prohibitions in his or her ethical code are simply ideals to be aspired to; failure to uphold these standards is seen as justified if one has made a "good effort." This approach can be seen as a form of rationalization for failure to exert the considerable self-discipline required to act in a professionally responsible manner.

It is also useful to note that ethical obligations leave a tremendous amount of latitude to the judgment of the practitioner. Perhaps this is as it should be because, as noted before, the nature of ethical behavior is that it be based in large part on the practitioner's *choices*. Further, the domains in which mental health practitioners claim expertise are ones which deeply affect the lives of those who call upon us for help. There are many ways to effectively help and a range of choices that respect individuals' personhood is available to the ethical clinician. It is finding one's way to such effective modes of practicing that the remainder of this book is devoted.

Chapter 2

A FRAMEWORK FOR ETHICAL DECISION MAKING

As we have suggested, no ethical practitioner (indeed no professional practitioner at all) can avoid making choices; the provision of ethically appropriate and clinically sound services requires constant and careful decision making. These deliberations about the ethically appropriate course of action may be excruciating in their detail, or quite fleeting, incorporated almost automatically into ongoing professional activities. The central ethical aspects of a particular problem may be immediately evident or extremely subtle, and the relevant professional standards may be clear-cut in their implications for action or frustratingly vague in providing guidance.

The purpose of this chapter is to present an explicit framework for ethical decision making. This framework is not intended to be rigorously followed each time an ethical question arises. Rather, it is an attempt to make explicit what should "naturally" occur in the course of deciding on an ethically appropriate action in practice. As we learn more about expertise in general, we find that highly skilled practitioners integrate an enormous amount of information in the context of underlying "operating principles" regularly in the course of their work (Patel & Groen, 1991). Generally, the practitioner's intuitive sense of the right decision (assuming proper training in competent professional service) will facilitate the decision-making process. However, as the ethical dimensions of practice become increasingly important and complex, attending to less obvious aspects of the decision-making process becomes vital.

In what follows, we briefly summarize the major "information gathering" aspects of the process of making ethical decisions; we then present a decision-making process and describe its possible uses.

PHASES OF INFORMATION GATHERING

This section describes three domains in which the practitioner must gather information before actually making a decision. Each area of information gathering can be conducted in more or less detail. One's information gathering may be as simple as mentally considering the relevant aspects of the situation, or it may be as complex as reviewing the literature, consulting with colleagues, and requesting professional opinions from philosophers, lawyers, or others. Briefly, the clinician must identify three elements before being able to make an ethical decision: (a) the nature of the ethical problem, (b) the identities and preferences of those persons who have a legitimate stake in the outcome of the problem (the "stakeholders"), and (c) the relevant professional and legal standards (if any) that bear on the case at hand. More detailed discussion of each of these domains follows.

Identifying the Ethical Problem

The first question in the initial analysis of a particular case is what makes this an ethical dilemma? Not all problems are ethical; some are simply technical. For example, a practitioner may wish to determine the best method for treating tension headaches. This is a technical decision and not (unless unusual circumstances exist) an ethical one. Conversely, deciding whether to inform the fiancée of a patient that her intended has episodic rage reactions *does* involve an ethical decision.

The key questions for the practitioner are first, is there an ethical problem or problems? Second, if more than one ethical problem exists, which is the most important? It is important to note with regard to this second issue that the tendency to proliferate dilemmas is always present. If at all possible, it is helpful to reduce the ethical dimensions of a situation to one or two primary ethical questions. Third, if an ethical dilemma can be identified, is there a way to resolve it without choosing between competing ethical principles? This is an important avenue in the initial decision-making process in that some ethical dilemmas can be reduced to technical problems by simply finding a method of operating that eliminates the conflict. For example, there is a potential conflict between the preservation of confidentiality when treating a minor client (e.g., an adolescent) and the legitimate demands of a worried parent to know what is happening in therapy. This can be a painful ethical dilemma, but therapists who work with children can routinely obtain permission from the parents of minors in advance (or at least discuss the issue openly before a crisis arises) so that this ethical dilemma does not arise so frequently.

Identifying Legitimate Stakeholders

In the typical hypothetical case (which almost never exists) the only parties legitimately concerned with the outcome of an ethical dilemma would be the practitioner and the client. In practice, however, other parties are typically involved. For example, often the party paying for mental health services is not the party receiving them. Such situations include cases in which the clinician is employed by an institution to render services, cases in which services are paid for by a third party, and cases in which a third party (such as an employer, parent, or court officer) legitimately orders professional services to be provided. In such cases, the clinician must clearly understand who has a legitimate right to be taken into account in making clinical decisions. The notion that some parties have legitimate stakes in the outcomes of a situation implies that their preferences about those outcomes should be taken into account. Once the identity of the stakeholders has been determined, some attempt to ascertain their preferences must be made.

In certain situations the problem is of such magnitude that parties not directly involved in contracting for the service have a legitimate stake in the outcome as well. In particular, it is at times essential to consider the interests of future members of the same class of consumer, unidentifiable members of society who may be affected by the outcome of the case, the practitioner's profession as a whole (and its image in the eyes of the public), and—most broadly—the general social climate in a particular society.

Thus, for example, decisions to breach or not to breach confidentiality may in part rest on considerations of the public's general level of trust in the mental health professions. Likewise, the decision to deceive or not to deceive a particular consumer about diagnosis or treatment plan may contribute to the general public distrust of professionals or a generally lowered level of respect for individuals in society.

Even though ethical decision making is sometimes presented as a purely cognitive or rational activity, it is important to recognize that there is a strong emotional or even aesthetic component to most ethical decisions. Ideally, such subjective preferences flow from a professional history of making ethical choices and carefully considering the contribution one's actions make to human welfare. Unfortunately, there can also arise situations in which a practitioner deduces from the applicable principles that a particular course of action is mandated but feels that it would not be "right" to engage in it. In such cases, reflection and consultation are called for. In the best outcome, either one's personal ethical standards or one's degree of comfort with sound ethical choices would evolve and mature.

Identifying Relevant Standards

Although we have until this point described the ethical dimension of professional decision making as almost entirely involving moral principles, society at large has taken intense interest in professional self-regulation. As a result, choices which might in the past have been made entirely on moral grounds ("Is this right or wrong?") are increasingly being made on mandatory grounds ("Is there a rule requiring or prohibiting this?"). Mental health practice, applied philosophy, and legal theory have become increasingly focused on the standards of practice as clients have shown their willingness to use legal power to enforce their view of appropriate professional actions. This in turn has led to the evolution of professional ethical codes into standards of practice. Precedents have emerged that mandate particular actions in particular situations. These precedents or standards may not always be clear-cut; however, once they exist in at least partially codified form, the responsible practitioner must have a good reason for *not* adhering to them. For example, the ethical mandate to obtain informed consent from patients has evolved into the expectation that clinicians will provide written information and obtain client signatures to indicate that the client has read and understood the information. On the other hand, the existing standards can be vague in their specifications for action. This does allow the practitioner to decide what the range of choices consistent with a given standard might be. For example, at the broadest level, the social workers' *Code of Ethics* (National Association of Social Workers, 1999) indicates in its Preamble that "The primary mission of the social work profession is to enhance human well-being and help meet the basic human needs of all people." The literal interpretation of this varies with the situation and with the specifics of the case.

An additional suggestion which may help in the identification of relevant standards is that one should not fear consultation in these matters. It is often unclear which, if any, existing professional standard bears on a specific case; consulting with experienced colleagues or experts in the particular area may help clarify the situation.

THE PROCESS OF ETHICAL DECISION MAKING

Once practitioners have gathered enough information to believe that they can adequately identify the ethical nature of the problems that face them, the legitimately involved parties, and the existing standards, they are in a position to begin to make a decision. This section describes a sequential process of establishing that an ethical decision has been made. It draws on a number of sources including material by Rest (1982), Jonsen, Siegler, and Winslade (1998), and Candee (1985). In the most general terms, this ethical decision-making framework rests on three underlying presumptions: the dignity and free will of the individual (autonomy), the obligation of professionals to respect the existing standards and expectations of the society that legitimizes their activities (responsibility), and the duty to avoid special or self-serving interpretations or situations (universality). In its simplest form the framework is presented as a flow chart in Figure 1 (page 12). Discussions of various phases of the flow chart follow.

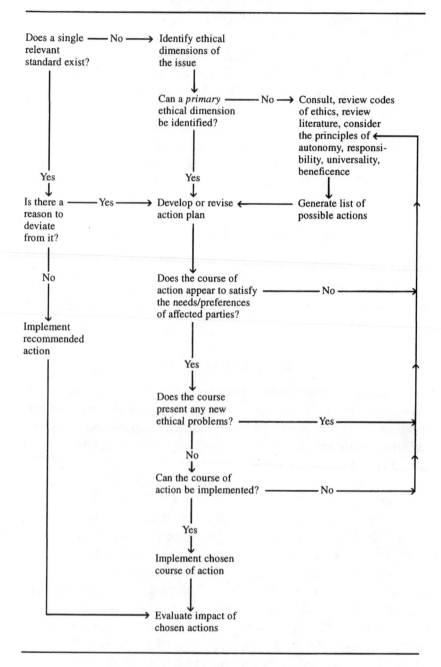

Figure 1. The Decision-Making Flow Chart.

Does a Relevant, Professional, Legal, or Social Standard Exist?

As implied in the preceding section, this question obligates the professional to engage in the common professional activity of literature review and/or consultation with respected colleagues. The nature of standards that may be accessed to answer this question range from the highly specific (e.g., *Standards for Educational and Psychological Testing* [American Educational Research Association et al., 1999] which mandate specific aspects of testing procedure) to the quite broad (e.g., the general social standard that one should keep one's promises, also codified in certain legal statutes that make fraud a criminal offense). As professional ethics codes and legal precedents evolve, there are fewer and fewer areas in which codified standards do not exist (see Committee on Professional Practice and Standards, 2003).

Is There a Reason to Deviate from the Standard?

Two types of cases may reduce the usefulness of existing standards. First, the existing standard may be so vague as to prevent its being used in a particular case. Second, the specifics of a given case may lead to more harm than benefit being produced by adhering to the standard (this is actually a special case of conflicting standards, because the overriding ethical obligation of all the mental health professions is to promote human welfare). An example of this question in use involves a case in which the mother of a 32-year-old patient being seen by a psychotherapist calls for information about her child.* A standard for this kind of case exists; the practitioner is obligated to uphold confidentiality. However, assume that in this case there is risk of suicide on the part of the patient. Then there may be a good reason to deviate from the professional standard in the interests of protecting patient welfare (however, note that this ethical dilemma may be resolved, if there is sufficient time, by contacting the patient and obtaining permission, even if it is not strictly required, before revealing information to the parent).

What Are the Ethical Dimensions of the Issue?

If there is no single ethical standard or principle which pertains,

---

*Names and all identifying characteristics of persons in all case examples have been disguised thoroughly to protect privacy.

the practitioner must identify the significant ethical issues. That is, what are the dimensions that make the issue problematic? For instance, is there a conflict between a need to preserve confidentiality and a need to protect the public? Mandatory child abuse reporting statutes frequently are used to illustrate this problem. On the one hand, it is argued that reporting suspected child abuse will drive out of treatment individuals who need it in order to parent their children effectively. On the other hand, it is argued that failure to report suspected abuse exposes the child in the family to the risk that the psychotherapist will not be able to affect the parents' acting out. The standard method of resolving this conflict involves the invocation of informed consent: The prospective client is informed at the outset of treatment that information regarding the possible abuse of a child must be reported. However, this solution raises another problem: Will the potentially abusive parent be encouraged to suppress information and thereby not get treatment for a significant problem? This presents a conflict between the obligation to honestly inform the prospective client about treatment and the obligation to provide competent service for the important problems. As another example, a clinical intervention which has been shown effective for a particular problem may be one that is rendered less effective the more the client knows about it (e.g., paradoxical intervention). Often, when the appropriate course of action is unclear, it is because of competing ethical principles; they must be defined and classified in order for there to be a chance to reconcile them.

Can a Primary Ethical Dimension be Specified?

When multiple ethical standards bear on a case, it is still often true that an overriding principle can be identified. For example, legal and ethical principles indicate that when clear and present danger exists, the obligation to protect potential victims overrides the obligation to uphold clients' understanding that the practitioner will keep information private. From a teleological perspective, this concept rests on the predictability of harm: The chances that harm will come to an individual who is being threatened by a potentially violent patient are greater than the chances that the patient will be harmed by the disclosure. Indeed, some commentators have suggested that truly benefiting potentially violent patients involves helping them to avoid acting on their violent impulses.

Consult and Review Codes of Ethics; Review Literature; Consider Ethical Principles

This implies that the practitioner has available resources (such as information, time, and energy) to review and extract usable information about ethical dilemmas. Other sections of this book will indicate possible resources that may help in this task, but it should be made clear that this task requires effort and diligence.

Generate a List of Possible Actions

In cases when no single ethical dimension outweighs all others, a variety of actions may prove to be ethically appropriate. As in other problem-solving situations, a "solution-generating" or "brainstorming" phase can be helpful. In this phase, the practitioner may benefit from reading relevant ethical codes, reviewing legal statutes, or consulting with colleagues. It is not always necessary to determine which ethical principle is dominant. Rather, time should be spent devising solutions which reconcile competing principles. Novel, creative solutions and ways to reconcile competing principles should be explored. For instance, in the case of the conflict between informed consent versus competence mentioned in connection with paradoxical therapy, the practitioner may be able to find a way to protect the client's right to know about treatment procedures without compromising the effectiveness of the intervention. Some authors have argued that this may be accomplished by providing some general information about treatment (appropriate to the client's level of sophistication) and allowing the client to ask for further information as needed. Others have argued that paradox works regardless of the level of awareness possessed by the client (Hunsley, 1988). Perhaps a treatment that relies on deception should be avoided unless there is a compelling need for it.

Following the brainstorming phase, a cost-benefit analysis should be conducted. Each alternative should be evaluated in terms of its potential benefits and potential costs. The needs of the client as well as the needs of other associated individuals (such as family members), the public, and the mental health profession should be considered. The alternative that results in an optimum resolution for the greatest number of interested parties should be chosen.

Does the New Course of Action Appear to
Satisfy the Needs/Preferences of Affected Parties?

While the ethical codes of all mental health disciplines underline the general obligation to promote human welfare, in particular cases this always translates into promoting the interests of one or more involved parties. Thus, if no standard exists with regard to a particular dilemma and/or there is good reason to deviate from existing standards because they seem inadequate to deal with the facts of the case, a course of action that takes into account (and, better yet, satisfies) the needs and/or preferences of affected parties must be developed. The notion here is that, all other things being equal, the practitioner is obliged to render the services which he or she has agreed to provide. Typically, the services are provided to satisfy some need of the consumer.

Does the Course of Action Present
Any New Ethical Problems?

This question is raised because of the nature of ethical decisions. Specifically, a major question that must be asked of any course of action to have it qualify as ethical is that of universalizability, as noted previously. In other words, would I recommend this same course of action to every other person essentially similar to me who is operating in essentially the same circumstances? This is a more limited version of this question: Would you recommend that everybody do this? This notion of universalizability is what distinguishes ethical action from expedient action. An example of this issue involves a case in which the patient of a psychotherapist is involved in a relationship the therapist considers extremely unhealthy. The therapist is in a position to be able to tell a "credible lie" to the patient regarding the behavior of her partner that would provoke her into leaving the relationship. The therapist believes that this action would be for the best interest of the patient. Is this an ethical course of action? We would argue that it is not, because the therapist could not reasonably expect that everyone in a similar situation should engage in a lie (thereby possibly reducing or damaging the trust the patient has in the therapist). Thus, the decision to lie would be seen as one of expediency rather than one of ethical responsibility. Another example involves the question of whether a clinician should accept a gift from a client. Assessing whether one would suggest the same course of action to other practitioners in the same situation clarifies the issue dramatically.

It is also a characteristic of ethical actions that they are based on principles. In the ideal case, the actor can specify the principles on which the course of action is based. A colloquial way of describing this element of the process has been proposed by D. Callahan (personal communication, 1980). It is the "clean, well-lit room" standard. That is, could the practitioner's decision be comfortably defended to a group of his or her peers in public? While some unethical decisions could pass this standard, no ethical decision should fail it.

Can the Course of Action be Implemented?

This question has two parts: It refers to issues of practicality and to issues of prudence. Practicality refers simply to the possibility that one could actually put the course of action into effect. Actions that involve social reform, changes in social policy, and massive upheavals in common ways of practice are unlikely to be implementable in a particular case. For example, suggesting to a depressed homemaker that she become more politically active and more conscious of her gender-based oppression would be considered (at least in the case of a patient who appears untroubled by her role choice) more likely to be a long-range political remedy rather than an implementable course of action.

The "prudence" aspect of this question refers simply to the fact that ethical decisions may at times be costly to the practitioner who implements them. Because effort and cost may be involved in implementing a decision, these issues should be thought through in advance. This sort of situation arises, for example, when a professional in training believes that a supervisor is acting unethically and wishes to confront him or her. While this may be the ethical course of action, it may also be professionally self-destructive. As we comment later, there are alternatives to an immediate confrontation that would be potentially less risky to one's training or career.

Implement the Chosen Course of Action

This recommendation appears straightforward but does involve other (nonethical) skills such as assertiveness, tenacity, the existence of a supportive social network, and the ability to communicate one's chosen action in noncondescending and humane terms. For example, psychologists are obligated to terminate a professional relationship when it is no longer beneficial to the consumer (American Psychological Association, 2002). It is sometimes the case that psychotherapists derive tremendous enjoyment from working with particular clients, and some clients, when confronted with the idea of termination, will resist and object to this. Nonetheless, despite the emotional difficulty of implementing such a decision, it may truly be the ethical course of action (in cases where no benefit but rather excessive client dependency seems to be developing) and may require technical expertise in communicating this decision to the client in a caring way.

Limitations of the Framework

A limitation inherent in this framework is that it is quite general. In later chapters, it will become clear that many specific situations have already been discussed, written about, and occasionally studied empirically. Although in these domains there may be fewer questions, no matter how much ethical theorizing and ethical research goes on, the continually evolving nature of professional practice will always produce cases with unique features that puzzle practitioners. The framework presented herein is simply to guide the practitioner in developing a perspective on such puzzling cases.

There are other limitations of this or any decision-making framework. Because a decision-making framework is based on rationality, there is no way to eliminate completely the possibility of self-serving rationalization. Additionally, the framework proposed above does not thoroughly take into account legal considerations. More generally, this may be considered as an issue of prudence. Is it prudent for a clinician to reason purely on the basis of ethical considerations without regard for legal liability or existing legal precedent? The answer is no. However, as a first step it is useful to consider the purely ethical or purely moral aspects of decision making. The prudential elements of the process can then be considered (as was briefly noted) under the question of implementability.

Finally, the proposed framework makes no allowances for ambiguity or mistakes. Certainly these occur, and it is in the nature of ethically responsible practice that one is not held blameworthy if one attempted to act appropriately and do what one thought was best. However, it is also ethically incumbent on the responsible practitioner to learn from his or her mistakes.

Chapter 3

COMPETENCE IN CLINICAL PRACTICE

The expectation that clinicians will deliver competent service is fundamental to the notion of professional mental health practice. This is borne out by the codes of ethics of the various mental health disciplines, which contain numerous statements focused on the issue of competence. For instance, the *Ethical Principles of Psychologists and Code of Conduct* (American Psychological Association, 2002) states, "Psychologists provide services, teach, and conduct research with populations and in areas only within the boundaries of their competence, based on their education, training, supervised experience, consultation, study, or professional experience" (Standard 2.01a). In a similar vein, "Counselors practice only within the boundaries of their competence, based on their education, training, supervised experience, state and national professional credentials, and appropriate professional experience" (American Counseling Association [ACA], 1995, § C.2.a).

The social workers' *Code of Ethics* (National Association of Social Workers [NASW], 1999) states, "Social workers continually strive to increase their professional knowledge and skills and to apply them in practice" (Competence Ethical Principle). The *Code of Ethics* of the American Association for Marriage and Family Therapy (AAMFT, 2001) asserts, "Marriage and family therapists pursue knowledge of new developments and maintain competence in marriage and family therapy through education, training, or supervised experience" (§ 3.1). *The Principles of Medi-*

cal Ethics With Annotations Especially Applicable to Psychiatry (American Psychiatric Association, 2001), states, "A physician shall be dedicated to providing competent medical service with compassion and respect for human dignity" (§ 1).

While the preceding statements, along with many others, underscore the importance of delivering competent service to patients or clients, defining what that competence consists of may be quite difficult.

Interestingly, at its root, competence is related to competition. Competence stems from the roots *com,* together, and *peter,* to seek: hence, to strive together or seek (Webster, 1956, p. 370). Consideration of the typical threshold for competent practice seems to rest on this aspect of the definition; that is, more clinicians than we would like to admit seem to consider themselves competent if they can match the abilities of "the competition." This might be considered the lowest common denominator standard for competence. Moving from a consideration of the roots of the term to its actual definition, however, shows that competence means "capacity equal to requirement; adequate fitness or ability" (Webster, 1956, p. 370). In law, competence is defined as "legal . . . qualification, . . . power, or fitness" to do something (Webster, 1956, p. 370). Thus, our analysis must focus on what it is that mental health practitioners are called upon to do. Also, professional competence includes both declarative expertise ("knowing what") and procedural expertise ("knowing how") (Faust, 1986).

Some might argue that attainment of competence occurs through obtaining the relevant credentials. Certainly credentials are necessary but not sufficient to establish professional competence. Credentials *per se* do not guarantee competence although presumably the lack of credentials would be a strong indicator of incompetence to perform certain professional activities.

It could also be inferred from the various professions' ethical codes that whenever practitioners violate an ethical principle, they can be said to have acted in an incompetent manner. Indeed, it may be asserted that *all* ethical principles can be derived from the principle of competence. Yet to define competence in this way makes the concept equivalent to the tenet of medical ethics, "above all, do no harm." While this is likely to generate little disagreement, it also leaves unenlightened the practitioner who wants to do some good (consistent with other tenets of all codes of professional ethics). Thus, this chapter discusses a more usable definition of competence, derived in part from concepts advanced by Wiens (1983), Haas (1993), Koocher and Keith-Spiegel (1998), and others.

Professional competence consists of appropriate professional education and training, continuing education, willingness to subject decisions to peer review, openness to criticism by colleagues, willingness to confess ignorance or error when appropriate, and concentrated and sustained efforts to deepen one's clinical craftsmanship (Pellegrino, 1979).

Stated differently, a competent clinician is one who has the requisite *knowledge* to understand and conceptualize a particular clinical issue, the necessary *skills* to apply this knowledge in effective ways, and the *judgment* to use such knowledge and skills. Put yet another way, the competent clinician knows what to do, how to do it, and when to do it. For example, a therapist who uses a heavily confrontational style of treatment with a prepsychotic individual may possess extensive knowledge about the technique but may lack judgment about the most appropriate situations in which to use it.

As this discussion implies, a major aspect of *professional* mental health practice is the moral obligation on the individual professional to ensure the quality of service. Currently, however, government (primarily at the state level), as the protector of potential patients, has become reluctant to rely solely on practitioners' ethics to guarantee competent treatment. Instead, for the purpose of protecting the public, legal standards of minimum competence have been established (and are constantly in the process of being refined). While this chapter deals in part with legal standards of minimum competence, our purpose is primarily to help the practitioner put the issue of competence into perspective in his or her own practice.

LICENSURE

The primary legal vehicle by which the public is protected from incompetent practice is licensure. While all states have provisions for the licensure or certification of at least some mental health professions, the question of the role of licensure in guaranteeing competent therapeutic service is nonetheless still hotly debated. The process has been criticized (e.g., Bernstein & LeComte, 1981;

Gross, 1978) and defended (e.g., Kane, 1982; Wiens, 1983) extensively in the literature. An extended discussion of licensure is beyond the scope of this book (cf. Fretz & Mills, 1980, for a review); however, there exist some issues regarding licensure that are relevant for the present discussion, and these are highlighted below.

Because the establishment of a professional relationship between a prospective patient and a clinician is a contractual matter, some practitioners might argue that the procedures are selected entirely at the choice of the contracting parties. That is, if the client or patient determines that the practitioner is competent enough for his or her purposes (and the practitioner agrees that he or she is competent to provide such services), that should be sufficient. Common examples of such assumptions include the following: (a) A community-organization trained social worker believes that licensing is a guild process and refuses to obtain a license. Nonetheless, he delivers services in a community agency which has full knowledge of the circumstances. (b) A second example is that of an industrial-organizational psychologist who believes that her work with individuals is not clinical service and refuses to obtain a license, and who provides occasional marital "advice" to consultees in the organization. (c) A third example is that of a marriage and family therapist who believes that the licensing examination in his profession is unfair and refuses to sit for it, holding himself out as a "mental health coach" and making it clear that no third-party reimbursement is possible for the services.

Despite the contractual nature of the relationship, a key assumption of the process of protecting the public is the notion that in the selection of professionals (be they accountants, psychotherapists, or electricians) the layperson is *not* able to adequately judge whether he or she is being well served. A full discussion of this debate is beyond the scope of this book; for further consideration of this issue as a public policy question, see Faden, Beauchamp, and King (1986). Regardless of the policy debates, from the perspective of protecting the public, the licensing process, however flawed, is justifiable. It is justifiable even though all that it can realistically signify is that an individual is able to demonstrate attainment of minimum levels of knowledge, education, and experience; it by no means guarantees competent or ethical practice. Given the practical, legal, and ethical questions raised, it is difficult to conceive of situations in which a practitioner who claims to deliver competent service is justified in not seeking the appropriate licensure or certification.

SELF-ASSESSMENT OF ONE'S OWN COMPETENCE

We assume the typical practitioner is usually well motivated and does not intentionally practice outside his or her area of professional competence. Nonetheless, it is likely that the cases involving competence heard by licensing boards, ethics committees, professional standards committees, and courts represent only a small fraction of those in which competence is an issue. The circumstances described below illustrate relevant points in this regard.

Example 1. A couple comes to a psychotherapist in private practice requesting sex therapy. The therapist has had no formal coursework in sex therapy but has read several of the major works in sex therapy and has attended a 2-day workshop on the subject. The therapist feels that he can probably help the couple. Can he consider himself competent to provide the requested service? Should his decision change if he has not read any of the major works in the area but has attended a workshop and has a knowledgeable colleague with whom he talks fairly often? Is he nonetheless competent to conduct sex therapy?

Example 2. A psychotherapist who has had considerable coursework and supervised experience in family therapy and who views herself as competent in this specialty is approached for treatment by a recently immigrated family. They are concerned about their teenage son and his failure to obey family rules. The therapist lives in an area in which there are few immigrant families, and this is the first immigrant family that she has worked with. Is she competent to deliver this type of service? Would this judgment change if she has worked with several immigrant families, but this is the first immigrant family she has worked with in which the son is receiving kidney dialysis? Is she still competent to deliver services?

The previous examples highlight some of the problems encountered in assessing one's competence. Although we have noted that a key component of competence is knowledge, how much knowledge is enough? Is one class enough? Is a 2-day workshop enough? Is reading a couple of books and talking to peers enough? Second, an important problem is that all clinical problems exist in particular contexts, and the context can dramatically change the requirements for competent service. The major issue here is defining what are general clinical principles that transcend particular contexts, and what are specific "micro-competencies" that are needed to deal effectively with unique client populations or circumstances. It is also important to remember that competence is not a static concept. Rather, it must be evaluated against the changing context of existing knowledge in the field. Thus, it is possible for one's competence to "erode" or "decay" over time. We discuss this further in Chapter 17.

These questions are not easily resolved. No credentialing body can possibly anticipate all possible situations a practitioner is likely to encounter and establish standards accordingly. Yet at the same time, the practitioner will be held responsible for delivering competent services even in the absence of such standards. While the decision-making process in such cases is of necessity abstract and ill-defined, listed below are five questions that one may find useful to consider in assessing his or her own competence to deal with a particular case. We assume that the practitioner is licensed in the profession for which he or she has been trained.

Guidelines for Assessing One's Competence

Is Your Approach Solidly Grounded in Research or Theory? A key feature that distinguishes mental health practice from religious approaches and faith healing is the emphasis on scientific evidence. Thus, the activities of the mental health professional are assumed to be grounded in the best available theory and research. When this notion is translated into the obligations for the individual provider, it becomes clear that the practitioner is obligated to be familiar with research and theoretical findings in the areas with which he or she deals.

This is somewhat easier said than done, however. Primarily, the reason for this difficulty is that there is a time lag between the point at which a critical mass of practitioners encounters a new problem, the point at which researchers can study the problem, and the point at which researchers can confidently recommend the optimum treatment of the problem. It is the nature of professional work that new problems are always emerging. Thus, the ethical practitioner should both search the literature to find what has gone before and should consider helping to create the emerging literature by reporting unusual cases or potential innovations in technique. Although this topic will be touched upon in Chapter 16, it is worth noting that from this perspective the research-and-publication enterprise takes on an ethical dimension.

Assuming that the practitioner is confronting a problem that is not rare or previously unheard of, it is important that each practitioner know where to access the existing data, even if those data were not part of his or her training originally. Thus, having access to professional information sources (particularly peer-reviewed journals) as well as to colleagues with relevant expertise is part of maintaining one's competence in a particular area. This notion adds an ethical dimension to the issue of obtaining continuing education and of preventing professional isolation.

Access to research may reveal contradictory findings in the literature. The research literature may contain conflicting recommendations or no obvious practical implications at all. This is often a problem that frustrated practitioners report when they attempt to derive implications for action from their readings of the scientific reports. This state of affairs increases the obligation on the practitioner to understand the limitations of empirical research in the mental health sciences but does not allow clinicians to simply ignore the research data as "irrelevant." For example, a therapist may be persuaded that aversion techniques hold great promise for treating habit disorders. However, reviewing the literature reveals many contradictory studies. Which ones are most relevant? In order to answer this question, the clinician must have (or be able to obtain) information about the appropriateness of the sample (e.g., Was the study conducted with college students or true agoraphobics?), the techniques employed (Was it "real" aversion as practiced in a clinical setting?), and the statistical analyses used (Was the effect big enough to be practically meaningful or only statistically significant because of a large sample size?). Competence at integrating the existing science with the clinical needs of one's patients is a key component of clinical excellence.

Competence has a legal dimension as well. Licensed practitioners can be held professionally liable for failing to deliver reasonably competent service. This is the basis for the malpractice claim of professional negligence. Legal authorities interpret "competent service" to mean having and using the knowledge, skill, and care ordinarily possessed and employed by members of the profession in good standing (Keeton, 1984). In the past, conforming to local custom (regardless of whether this was in keeping with current findings) was held to protect the practitioner from findings of negligence (King, 1986). However, local standards of practice have essentially given way to national standards. It is assumed that all practitioners now have access to sources of information that would allow them to stay current with nationally emerging findings.

Do Relevant Standards Exist? Treatment guidelines for various disorders, as opposed to training standards for the application of various techniques, are increasingly prevalent. Such efforts have been sponsored and endorsed by a variety of mainstream professional associations, not simply the more specialized organizations or societies. For instance, the American Psychiatric Association, the American Psychological Association, and the National Association of Social Workers have all developed various practice guidelines (many available on their web pages), covering such far-ranging topics as guidelines for psychological evaluations in child protection matters, standards of practice for social work mediators, and practice guidelines for the psychiatric evaluation of adults.

In addition, manuals and protocols for evidence-based or empirically supported treatment of various disorders are being developed at a rapid rate from numerous sources. These manuals are often very specific in the steps that are to be taken in the treatment of such disorders and problems as borderline personality disorder, panic disorder, and poor anger management.

From both ethical and practical perspectives, there is considerable difference of opinion regarding the application of such structured treatment approaches. While there is an obvious benefit to the application of empirically validated treatments, there is also concern about whether the structure provided by such guidelines can adequately take into account the variability of individuals with a certain disorder. For example, following the manual's directions for treatment of panic disorder may result in an approach that ignores crucial characteristics of a given individual with that disorder. We believe that the clinician must use his or her judgment in each case. These concerns are especially relevant when a third party (e.g., an HMO or insurance plan) insists that all participating clinicians follow a particular treatment protocol to obtain reimbursement.

Another version of the problem was highlighted in a recent seminar on the treatment of borderline personality disorders. This seminar focused on a manual-based treatment with considerable research support. A participant raised his hand and asked why, given his vast clinical experience, he should be so limited in his approach. The presenter responded that if she ever had to go to court to defend herself in a malpractice action, she considered her adherence to the manual to be her best defense.

Another emerging concern relates to the problem of conflicting guidelines. As manual-based treatment, preferred practice guidelines, treatment protocols, and the like proliferate, they may very well result in contradictory recommendations. The American Psychiatric Association (1997) sought guidance on this question from the federal Agency for Health Care Policy and Research (now known as the Agency for Health Research and Quality). Recommendations for dealing with contradictory guidelines included asking the following questions:

1. Who sponsored the guidelines? Where did the money come from?
2. How recent are the data on which they were based?
3. What methodology was used? How did [the authors] go about doing what they did? Was it based on evidence? What was the evidence? Was the methodology specific? Did they lay out ahead of time what they were going to do? What population was the work normed on?
4. Are the treatments suggested by the practice guidelines affordable and accessible? Or are they so onerous that no one could ever use them?
5. How were the guidelines reviewed, and how do they relate to other practice guidelines?

The ethical implications of structured or standardized approaches to treatment are evolving. Nonetheless, practitioners will increasingly need to demonstrate awareness of relevant guidelines and empirically validated treatments for the disorders they treat and to justify deviations from these guidelines. Potentially, inability to demonstrate such awareness may be considered an ethical violation.

What Contextual Constraints Apply? Just as clinical problems are always nested in a particular context, so is clinical competence dependent on *its* context. For instance, whether a particular clinician should be considered capable of handling a particular case has some relationship to other services available to the client. In a small community with only a handful of therapists, the *only* alternative to accepting a wide range of cases may be to deny treatment to patients (and to commit professional suicide). In more urban settings, the failure to refer to better-trained specialists (and subspecialists) may be to risk malpractice actions (and professional suicide). The *client's* perception of alternatives is also relevant in this regard. If a therapist believes that the client may not continue with treatment if referred to a specialist, then the option of working with the client (and perhaps obtaining consultation) becomes more defensible.

It is often the case that an individual working in an institutional setting is expected to pick up cases as assigned. In such environments, refusing clients because of self-perceived inability to deal with the presenting problems may be impractical or politically unwise. The practitioner in such cases has an increased responsibility to obtain appropriate inservice training, supervision, or continuing education of some sort to provide the best treatment to the patient. However, the clinician should not silently submit to such work conditions. In fact, organizations that insist that clinical staff take on cases they may be ill-prepared for while at the same time denying them needed support are setting the stage for clinical burnout and patient neglect.

Are You Emotionally Able to Help the Client? In addition to deficits in skills or knowledge, competence can be diminished in a number of other ways. These include such problems as counter-transference, personal preoccupations, transient stress, "engagement" (Beier & Young, 1984) with the client, stereotyping, and the like. These difficulties present technical as well as ethical issues because recognizing them and overcoming them are part of what it means to be a competent psychotherapist.

For example, the psychotherapist who is recently divorced may be at special risk for introducing distortions into an otherwise competent treatment process; the workaholic therapist who finds himself or herself drowsy or irritable during sessions may be at risk for damaging the working relationship or of missing important therapeutic information. These are simply two examples of ways in which the therapist's difficulties (not necessarily resulting from skill or knowledge deficits) may intrude on competent treatment. Clearly, therapists are human and must learn to recognize their human limitations.

The implications of the foregoing are that therapists should (a) have the ability to monitor themselves accurately, (b) have available consultants to whom they can turn for expert advice and for feedback on their own behavior, (c) have social support networks that can provide "resources" in times of stress and that can help prevent them from becoming "depleted," (d) consider personal therapy (this point may seem obvious, but it is remarkable to us how much resistance there seems to be among mental health practitioners to obtaining personal therapy), (e) have available or consider developing referral sources to whom they can send cases beyond their competence, and (f) have the self-discipline and integrity to limit their practices to those cases with which they can deal competently.

Can the therapist assume that he or she will naturally become aware of impaired functioning? We believe that ordinary human defenses of rationalization and suppression operate all too easily among psychotherapists; thus, clinicians should consciously monitor the existence of such conditions. Seeking feedback from trusted associates (and receiving this feedback nondefensively) is of utmost importance in recognizing and correcting potentially disabling conditions.

The incompetent or less-than-competent senior practitioner may be "burned out" (G. Corey, M. S. Corey, & Callanan, 1988) or impaired as a result of psychopathology or substance abuse (Haas & Hall, 1990). Burned-out professionals are characterized by negative attitudes toward themselves, others, work, and life (G. Corey et al., 1988) and may experience a sense of fragmentation stemming from having attempted to do too many professional activities at the same time. Sadly, both burned-out and impaired professionals sometimes have extreme difficulty becoming aware of their limitations, and forceful confrontation by concerned colleagues is often necessary.

Could You Justify Your Decision to a Group of Your Peers? The "clean, well-lit room" standard can prove very useful in making decisions about one's competence to handle a particular situation. That is, the clinician should be aware of prevailing clinical standards and practices, and if deviating from them, ask himself or herself how that might be justified. Because there is very little scrutiny of the vast majority of treatment decisions made by practitioners, it is easy to become casual and lose sight of appropriate standards, making decisions that are significantly at variance with common practices. This speaks to the importance of maintaining active contacts and involvements in one's professional community. It also speaks to the importance of making decisions with current standards of practice in mind. Clinical problems are so varied that many different approaches are acceptable, but underlying these specific approaches is a set of values (some standards of competence included) to which each mental health profession ascribes. Even when working independently, a therapist would do well to ask himself or herself such questions as whether the decisions being made would be the same if a panel of peers were present, and whether the clinician would recommend the same course of action to others.

Chapter 4

PRIVACY, CONFIDENTIALITY, AND PRIVILEGE

The closely linked concepts of privacy, confidentiality, and privilege are crucial components of effective clinical practice. Together they represent the guarantee of trustworthiness and safekeeping—legal, professional, and moral—that the psychotherapist offers to the client. While empirical data on this issue are sparse, the available evidence (DeKraii & Sales, 1984; Gomes-Schwartz, Hadley, & Strupp, 1978) points out that trust is essential to effective clinical work. Why is this so? The process of psychotherapy typically requires that a client explore and discuss with the therapist information that may be intimate, sensitive, and often painful for the client to acknowledge even to himself or herself. How can we ask a client to trust us enough to share such information if we can't ensure that it will remain the individual's own information, to be shared with others at his or her own discretion?

With this in mind, it is essential that clients understand the protections granted to them in the clinical context, and it is essential that clinicians understand their ethical obligation to protect the confidentiality of clinical information and their legal obligation to respect privileged communications. Further, it is critical that clients and clinicians also know the limits of confidentiality and privilege rights.

This chapter addresses the nature of the interrelated concepts of privacy, confidentiality, and privilege. It discusses some of the limits to confidentiality that the practitioner is likely to encounter. Finally, summary guidelines will be presented to aid the practitioner in decision making about breaching confidentiality.

PRIVACY

The "right to privacy" is a general philosophical concept embedded in a Western view of human dignity (Caplan, 1982). Basically, the notion that individuals have a right to privacy implies that human autonomy carries with it the privilege of keeping secrets. That is, information about oneself should be one's possession, to be dispensed at one's discretion. Elements of a "right to privacy" can be found in the *Bill of Rights of the United States Constitution,* for example, the right of citizens to be "secure in their persons, house, papers and effects" (Webster, 1956/US Constitution, 4th Amendment), as well as in many other legal precedents. It is a deeply ingrained belief in American society that individuals have a right to keep information about themselves private.

Confidentiality and privilege, to be described below, can be looked at as derivatives of the right to privacy. Both concepts are justified by the general philosophical belief that individuals have a right to keep information about themselves private, and by the psychological truth that "exposure" of private information to others can result in psychic and other kinds of damage.

CONFIDENTIALITY

Confidentiality is professional privacy. Information has been shared with another, and that other has the duty to keep private information private. The obligation to uphold confidentiality is a key component of the ethical codes of all mental health professions. For example, psychologists' *Ethical Principles of Psychologists and Code of Conduct* (American Psychological Association, 2002) states, "Psychologists have a primary obligation and take reasonable precautions to protect confidential information obtained through or stored in any medium, recognizing that the extent and limits of confidentiality may be regulated by law or established by institutional rules or professional or scientific relationship" (Standard 4.01). The psychiatrists' code notes that "Confidentiality is essential to psychiatric treatment" (American Psychiatric Association, 2001, § 4). Social workers are urged to "protect the confidentiality of all information obtained in the course of professional service, except for compelling professional reasons" (NASW, 1999, § 1.07c). Marriage and family therapists "have unique confidentiality concerns because the client in a therapeutic relationship may be more than one person. Therapists respect and guard the confidences of each individual client" (AAMFT, 2001, Principle II). Counselors "respect their clients right to privacy and avoid illegal and unwarranted disclosures of confidential information" (ACA, 1995, § B.1.a).

Maintaining client confidences protects more than just the particular client-therapist relationship. It also protects the public trust in the mental health professions more generally. If practitioners are perceived to be "loose-lipped" (e.g., as a result of being heard discussing their clients), clients or prospective clients may be inhibited in discussing sensitive matters.

In addition to the ethical dimension of confidentiality, there are some legal issues which bear mentioning. First, licensing statutes frequently incorporate the profession's ethical standards into their language. This makes the licensed practitioner legally bound to uphold confidentiality. Second, legal precedents regarding what constitutes usual and customary treatment (DeKraii & Sales, 1984) may well put the practitioner who breaches confidentiality at legal risk even in the absence of a specific statute.

PRIVILEGE

Privileged communications are related to admissions in court testimony, as opposed to confidentiality, which deals with all communications (see Knapp & VandeCreek, 1987). The concept of privilege is a legal rather than an ethical one (Cohen & Mariano, 1982). Specifically, privilege statutes grant patients of certain clinicians the right to prevent the clinician from revealing information in a court proceeding. Such privilege statutes indicate that the state's legislative bodies consider the preservation of the trust relationship between clinician and client to be more important than the need of the courts to have access to all information potentially usable as evidence.

One additional distinction between privilege and confidentiality is that privilege is a legally guaranteed right of the patient whereas confidentiality is an ethical obligation of the service provider. It must be noted that privilege can be waived by the client, but not by the professional (Schwartz, 1989). That is, the clinician does not have the right to reveal privileged information against the client's wishes (unless ordered to do so by the court), nor does the clinician have the right to maintain that communications are privileged if the client waives privilege.

Privilege is not granted to all mental health professionals. State statutes vary in terms of the classes of practitioners to whom privilege is granted. Clinicians should consult local statutes in order to determine whether client communication is privileged. The status of privilege in federal courts has changed dramatically following the U.S. Supreme Court's decision in the *Jaffee v. Redmond* case (1996). Prior to this decision, psychotherapist-patient privilege was not granted as a general matter in federal cases. However, in *Jaffee v. Redmond,* the court acknowledged the importance of psychotherapist-client privilege. This case, and subsequent decisions, indicate that support for the concept of privilege is quite strong in the federal system. However, because the application of privilege continues to be refined and further defined in judicial decisions, the practitioner would be well advised to seek legal consultation when being ordered to reveal client information in federal courts.

It must also be noted that privilege is not absolute. It may be qualified by state law, as in cases of suspected child abuse. In fact, in any judicial proceeding, judges are the ultimate interpreters of when and how privilege applies, and judges seem to differ in terms of the extent to which they honor privilege. Despite this, it is very important that clinicians not be too hasty in revealing privileged information. They should honor the client's privilege until clearly ordered not to do so by the court (Committee on Professional Practice and Standards, 2003).

COMPLICATED CONFIDENTIALITY SITUATIONS

The existence of ethical mandates and legal rulings still leaves many difficult confidentiality decisions in the hands of the professional. Clearly, protecting confidentiality is important, but it should be kept in mind that confidentiality is not an end in itself; rather, it is a means to the end of effective, responsible, caring treatment of patients' emotional or behavioral difficulties. In this section we focus on a number of complicated situations in which other demands impinge on the mental health professional that may affect the decision whether to breach or protect confidentiality. This discussion does not include consideration of routine requests for information from other professionals or third-party payors for which the client has voluntarily given permission; such situations do not typically represent an ethical question or dilemma. Circumstances to be considered are as follows:

1. Health Insurance Portability and Accountability Act of 1996 (HIPAA) considerations
2. Court subpoenas
3. Duty to warn, protect, or report
4. Requests for information from family members
5. Custody issues
6. Group treatment
7. Difficulty defining the client
8. Multiple staff in an agency
9. Professional needs (consultation, teaching, support)
10. Managed care requirements

HIPAA CONSIDERATIONS

We include HIPAA (P.L. 104-191) considerations for two reasons: First, HIPAA is a very complicated piece of legislation that effectively applies to all mental health practitioners, and it applies in conjunction with state law (e.g., state regulations that are more stringent in a particular area take precedence). Second, if patients object to the sharing of information, as they are permitted to do, HIPAA can challenge the practitioner's ability to balance legal and ethical responsibilities.

HIPAA provides that all clinicians involved in the treatment of a patient (subsumed under the category "covered entities") can share protected health information (PHI) about that individual as long as he or she has been given the opportunity to object to this sharing. However, professionals do not have to agree to the patient's request (see recommendations below). In addition, information may be shared with covered entities involved with payment and health care operations. Health care operations are defined as administrative, financial, legal, and quality improvement activities such as peer reviews and audits (Office of Civil Rights, 2003). Assuming that the patient has had the opportunity to object, HIPAA also allows a health care provider to "disclose to a family member, other relatives, or a close personal friend of the individual, or any other person identified by the individual, the protected health information directly relevant to such person's involvement with the individual's care or payment related to the individual's health care" (P.L. 104-191, § 164.510 (b)(1)(i)).

Psychotherapy notes are excluded from the information that may be released without the patient's specific authorization. The definition of "psychotherapy notes" is quite specific and narrow, as noted in Chapter 10. Regardless of the reason for releasing protected health information, HIPAA rules specify that only the minimum necessary information can be released.

Our belief is that, despite the specificity of HIPAA standards, there remain many areas of ethical discretion. Below are some suggestions for making ethical decisions within HIPAA guidelines:

1. Given the complexities of HIPAA, the ethical mandate is to tailor the level of detail to the client's level of understanding. All that is technically required is that you provide the individual with a copy of your privacy practices; ethically, you may often need to do much more and clearly indicate what the patient has the right to request that you restrict.

2. If the patient does object to disclosure and you believe that you cannot deliver appropriate services under the requested restrictions, then it is appropriate to either deny the request or discontinue treatment.

3. Use professional judgment in deciding what information meets the definition of "minimum necessary."

4. Be deliberate in decisions regarding the involvement of family members. Although HIPAA increases clinicians' abilities to share information with patients' families, those decisions still require careful professional judgment.

5. "Verify" the identity of the individual with whom you are sharing information. In an actual situation known to one of us (JLM), a patient's ex-husband called for information about her treatment claiming to be her internist.

The HIPAA privacy regulations can safeguard patient privacy rights while allowing health care providers to deliver services in an effective and efficient manner without undue encumbrances.

As noted, HIPAA is complex, and additional resources, such as the Office of Civil Rights (2003) report can be useful.

Court Subpoenas

The receipt of a subpoena, despite its official nature, does not mean that the practitioner must immediately release whatever information is requested (this point will be discussed further in Chapter 10). On the other hand, it is obviously unwise to rely on the fact that one has the statutory protection of privilege and refuse to respond to a court order. As noted earlier, regardless of state statutes to the contrary, judges may feel that it is within their power to insist on disclosure of information in particular court cases (Cohen & Mariano, 1982). The judge's authority to find a professional in contempt of court is important to remember in this regard. Also, since the client "owns" the privilege, the decision to waive privilege or insist upon it should heavily weight the client's wishes. This fact does not absolve the professional of ethical responsibility to advise the client about the potential risks of disclosure, however. It may also be ethically proper to consider negotiating less damaging alternatives to revealing information in open court. Options may include holding a private meeting in the judge's chambers or providing written summary from the therapist to be released to both attorneys and to the judge.

If the client does not waive privilege, then the prudent course for the professional to follow is to obtain legal consultation (Bennett et al., 1990). Such issues as the nature of the subpoena, relevant privilege statutes, the desires of the client, and possible negative consequences of revealing the information are relevant and, unless very familiar to the practitioner, should be clarified with legal help. If the client has an attorney, it is wise to consult with this person as well.

Duty to Warn, Protect, or Report

Initially crystallized as legal precedent by the now-famous *Tarasoff* decision (*Tarasoff v. Board of Regents of the University of California,* 1976), the duty to protect mandates that when practitioners become aware of a threat of physical harm posed by their patient or client to an identifiable individual or individuals, they incur a duty to take some action to protect the intended victim. While earlier interpretations by many clinicians translated this obligation as a "duty to warn" (Bersoff, 1976), it is more accurate to describe the legal obligation as a "duty to protect" (VandeCreek & Knapp, 2001). As described in Chapter 7, this latter interpretation (unless superseded by local state court rulings or statutes) gives the practitioner more options in deciding what actions may be taken.

The duty to report is similar to the duty to protect and is based on belief that certain conditions are considered by the state to be so dangerous, either to the public welfare or to specific individuals, that reports of their existence must be made regardless of the potential harm to the treatment process. The duty to report is, in theory, simpler to discharge than duties to warn or protect, in the sense that the duty is typically discharged by a phone call to the proper authorities.

The most notable example of the duty to report, embodied in the statutes of all 50 states (Butz, 1985; VandeCreek & Knapp, 2001), is the duty to report suspected child abuse. Additionally, many states have also passed mandatory reporting statutes for "vulnerable adults and elderly populations," as well (Bergeron & Gray, 2003). While this duty is incumbent on any citizen, it has been explicitly extended to cover health care professionals (as well as teachers and social service workers), in that practitioners are in an extremely good position to detect evidence of possible abuse. Although substantial numbers of practitioners violate these statutes (Kalichman & Craig, 1991), clinicians who do so place themselves in an extremely vulnerable position. From a legal perspective, the nonreporting clinician has decided to violate the law, presumably in favor of some more valued outcome such as maintaining a productive treatment relationship, or perhaps because of doubts about the usefulness of reporting and the wish to spare the family this difficulty. From an ethical perspective, the nonreporting clinician has decided that continued treatment without reporting is in the best interests of the child and the parent(s) and has thus taken on greater responsibility for ensuring that treatment does indeed improve the parent's ability to master his or her acting out. The problem with almost all of the statutes is that they mandate reporting on suspicion of abuse, and thus the psychotherapist may be reluctant to involve the family in a child abuse investigation on the basis of suspected problems; on the other hand, the therapist is himself or herself liable to prosecution if a district attorney decides that the suspicion should have reached the threshold for reporting (VandeCreek & Knapp, 2001). The prudent clinician will know what the definition of abuse is in the state in which he or she practices because definitions differ. He or she will also have thought through (preferably in advance, and possibly with the client directly) what the steps in reporting should be. For example, it is sometimes recommended that helping a parent to report directly is preferable (in terms of their later treatment by the child-protection agency) than to have the professional report (VandeCreek & Knapp, 2001).

AIDS and HIV create special legal and ethical challenges in this regard. The number of individuals infected with the HIV virus, the spread of this virus, and the devastating effects of AIDS have created ethical dilemmas for clinicians who work with HIV-infected clients. In many respects these dilemmas are similar to those posed by potentially violent or potentially abusive clients (Huprich, Fuller, & Schneider, 2003).

Although any sexually transmitted disease raises the issue of risks to which an unwitting sexual partner is exposed, the incurable and fatal nature of HIV infection has brought to the forefront of clinicians' consciousness the dangers faced by sexual partners of their HIV-positive clients. This realization may force clinicians to balance several issues: the presenting issue that brings the client to treatment (often it is not the issue of how to ensure that they keep partners safe from HIV infection), the maintenance of a productive therapy relationship, improving the clients' ability to confront and resolve the problems revealed by their failure to inform a partner or to practice safe sex, and the duty (if any) to protect the well-being of ignorant sexual partners.

It is important to note in this regard that a substantial number of HIV-positive individuals do not intend to reveal their serostatus to sexual partners (Kegeles, Catania, & Coates, 1988). An example may illuminate some of the issues. A psychotherapist sees a young woman who has recently discovered that she tests positive for HIV, which she presumably contracted through her intravenous use of drugs. She has one primary sexual partner and several occasional sexual partners. She has not told any of them that she tests positive. The clinician would be permitted, but not required, to report her condition to her partners. However, to do so might seriously impair the quality of the therapeutic relationship. The result of reporting might be that the present partners may be protected, but the client may leave treatment prematurely, thus preventing her from resolving whatever psychological conflicts led her to keep this information from them in the first place and possibly endangering future sexual partners. Thus, it is probably clinically wiser, at least as a first step, to discuss the issue and help the client see the wisdom of revealing her condition to her partners herself. Current case law does not suggest that the therapist is liable should the woman infect a partner, but case law continually changes.

There are many variations in the types of situations with which a clinician is confronted in working with HIV-positive patients; therefore, the appropriate course of action may vary (Erickson, 1990). It is generally preferable to handle these situations within a clinical context and with the client's cooperation. However, there are several additional factors that are relevant. First, a number of states have enacted laws pertaining to HIV infection (Macklin, 1991). The precedent for reporting (to health authorities, at least) that one's patient has an infectious disease is long established in medicine. Second, standards have been developed by various mental health organizations which leave considerable professional discretion to the clinician. As noted, a substantial portion of HIV-infected individuals will not reveal to their sexual partners, especially nonprimary partners, that they are infected (Knapp & VandeCreek, 1990). There are ambiguities in the situation: In what sense is the sexual partner identifiable to the therapist? Is there a moral obligation either way, absent a legal obligation, to report or to maintain confidentiality? Is there foreseeable harm (the standard established in *Tarasoff*-like decisions)? Knapp and VandeCreek (1990), in an interesting discussion of this problem, suggest that it is incumbent upon therapists who have HIV-positive clients to ascertain how much risk they are placing on their patients' partners, as different sexual practices entail differing degrees of risk. Most likely, the therapist will have to face these issues even if the HIV status of the patient is unknown (especially if the patient engages in high-risk behavior and refuses to get tested). Position statements by the American Psychological Association and the American Psychiatric Association place the burden on the therapist, indicating that it is not required—but is also not prohibited—to break confidentiality when danger is imminent. Other sources of information (e.g., Beck, 1982) suggest that openness about the risks the patient is running, and openness about the need to allow the partner to make an informed decision, can actually result in better outcomes (e.g., patient or therapist does disclose, harm is prevented, and treatment continues).

Requests for Information from Family Members

Often, for more or less pressing reasons, members of a client's family will contact the clinician and reveal or request information. Although the most common cases concern parents inquiring about their children's treatment, difficult ethical questions arise for the practitioner whether the confidentiality issue concerns a child or an adult. Each of these circumstances will be described below.

When the Client Is a Child. Does a child have a right to confidentiality? Legally, no. In most cases, the parents as the legal guardians responsible for the child have the right to know what is going on in treatment. In fact, if the parent does not protect the child's well-being, he or she is vulnerable to charges of child neglect. It is important for the practitioner to be sensitive to the parents' legal obligation to know what is going on in treatment, as well as to the parent's emotional concerns for the child.

On the other hand, regardless of the legalities, it may be desirable from a practical or ethical perspective to offer the child the same assurances of confidentiality that would be offered to an adult. Technically, to do this, the parent must waive his or her rights of access to the information. It is obviously much better to negotiate this permission before treatment begins rather than trying to negotiate it in the heat of a crisis. Ideally, both child and parent should know under what circumstances (e.g., life-threatening situations) confidential information will be revealed.

When the Client Is an Adult. Family members often feel that they have a right to know what is going on in treatment with a family member (e.g., "I'm her husband, and she should have no secrets from me"). Although an adult client in individual treatment has rights of confidentiality even with respect to other family members, the situation becomes more complicated when the practitioner is working with a couple or a family and sees the clients together at times and separately at others. If a client reveals information in an individual session, should another family member have access to that information? If the family is clearly the "client," then a case could be made that revealing such information would be ethically justified. However, based on assumptions about the principle of confidentiality, a client may assume the confidentiality is extended to individuals, not systems. Thus, he or she could reasonably expect that information shared with the clinician individually is confidential, even if other family members are being seen. Despite the view among systems theorists that the family is the "client," ethics codes clearly suggest that the right of confidentiality belongs to the invididual and not the family. Marriage and family therapists "respect and guard the confidences of each individual client" (AAMFT, 2001, Principle II). The *Code of Ethics* of the American Counseling Association also makes a clear statement regarding this: "In family counseling, information about one family member cannot be disclosed to another member without permission. Counselors protect the privacy rights of each family member" (ACA, 1995, § B.2.b).

These statements appear to suggest that, at least for the disciplines involved, the practitioner does not have a right to decide whether to share information given to him or her in "secret" by a family member. This places a serious burden on the practitioner to anticipate the possibility of receiving unwanted information so that he or she can respond in an appropriate manner, possibly by stopping the family member from sharing the information in the first place.

An issue which has been receiving increased attention relates to the question of the confidentiality of an adult who is severely mentally ill and whose family members request information. Various individuals and advocacy groups have complained that clinicians are too stringent in their interpretations of confidentiality rights as they apply to families of schizophrenic and other mentally ill adults. Specifically, they are concerned that professionals share too little information with the family members, who often are the primary caregivers of these individuals (Petrila & Sadoff, 1992).

There are many considerations which must be raised in resolving questions about whether to reveal information to the family of a mentally ill client. The first relates to the clinician's own attitudes. As an example, we are aware of situations in which a clinician has refused to give information to the family of a schizophrenic client, citing confidentiality as the reason, when he did not even bother to ask the patient what she wanted to have done. It is important that confidentiality not be used as a smoke screen for personal convenience.

It is our belief that if the family of a mentally ill patient requests information, the clinician consults the client, and the client refuses to grant permission, then this refusal must ordinarily be honored even if the refusal is based on some type of delusional thinking. That is, the presence of a mental illness does not necessarily remove an individual's civil rights, including the right to confidentiality. The exception to this, in our estimation, is when there is a reason to believe that the client is unable to take care of himself or herself and needs someone to act in his or her behalf. For instance, a psychotic client in the midst of an acute exacerbation of symptoms may need to be involuntarily committed, and it is appropriate to seek the family's assistance in this matter. It should go without saying that in cases in which ethical standards demand the refusal of information to the family, clinical sensitivity is essential. The family remains a potential partner to the clinician in caring for the patient with serious mental illness.

Custody Issues

Not infrequently, after marital or family (or even individual) treatment has been delivered, families dissolve. If a custody battle ensues, one or the other partner may subpoena the practitioner for the treatment records. In such cases the practitioner may have few legal grounds on which to resist a subpoena. Although practitioners may believe that they are protected by privileged-communication statutes, Knapp and VandeCreek (1987) cite several ways in which courts may override patient-therapist privilege when the interests of a child are at stake in a custody dispute. Nonetheless, if pretreatment agreements can be negotiated that prevent one member of the couple from subpoenaing information without the consent of the other member, the clinician may possibly be on firmer ground. Although the pretreatment arrangement is probably not legally binding, it may dissuade parties from seeking the notes from conjoint therapy.

Direction in releasing such information is provided by the AAMFT *Code of Ethics* (AAMFT, 2001) as it states "When providing couple, family or group treatment, the therapist does not dis-

close information outside the treatment context without a written
authorization from each individual competent to execute a waiver.
In the context of couple, family or group treatment, the therapist
may not reveal any individual's confidences to others in the
client unit without the prior written permission of that individual"
(§ 2.2).

From the ethical point of view, practitioners must do what is
in the best interest of the client. But, in this case, who is the client?
Some practitioners take the position that they will provide no
testimony in future divorce or custody actions once they have
seen a couple together. Others, who have seen only one member
of the couple, may find that it is inappropriate for them to testify
unless they have had direct contact with the other member of the
marital pair. Clearly, the most advantageous position is to negotiate or at least think through these issues beforehand. It is also important in custody cases to distinguish between the role of expert
witness (who may be entitled to give an opinion on the relative
fitness of each of the parents) and the role of fact witness (who is
restricted to reporting what he or she has observed). The difficulties encountered by therapists who submit to subpoena by one
party when they have seen both partners or who agree to testify
as evaluators when they have functioned as therapists are significant and best avoided if possible (Haas, 1993).

Group Treatment

The practice of group psychotherapy places a unique confidentiality demand on the clinician. Information shared in group
therapy can be just as sensitive and personal as it is in individual
therapy, but other clients who do not share the clinician's obligation to protect confidentiality become privy to the information. The
practitioner has an obligation to take whatever steps are possible
to safeguard the confidentiality of the information shared in groups.
At the very least, the group members' responsibility to keep information confidential should be emphasized during the first session,
and this should be reiterated as often as needed (e.g., when new
members join the group, or when a member feels vulnerable about
something that has been shared). Also, the practitioner might
consider making himself or herself available to see a client individually to deal with very sensitive information. In the course of
such an individual session, the practitioner could discuss the mat-

ter with the client and decide together whether it should be shared with other group members. This alternative may be unacceptable to practitioners who hold firmly to the rule that there should be no secrets from other group members, but such practitioners may have an added responsibility to ensure confidentiality within the group. The use of written contracts signed by group therapy participants has been advocated as well.

Difficulty Defining the Client

At times it may be unclear who the client is. For instance, if a practitioner is hired by the correctional system to provide psychotherapy for prison inmates or provides treatment services to those in military service, there are questions regarding what guarantees of confidentiality can be provided to the patients. The preferred solution is to anticipate potential problems and negotiate and agree on solutions before treatment begins. This issue is described in greater depth in Chapter 8.

Multiple Staff in an Agency

There may be a difference in the assumptions made by a practitioner and a client concerning information to be shared with other staff members in an agency. The practitioner may assume that the guarantee of confidentiality to the client still allows the case to be openly discussed with other agency personnel. The client, on the other hand, may assume that the guarantee of confidentiality means that the information will be discussed with no one else. The various codes of ethics seem to favor the client's point of view. That is, the obligation of confidentiality seems to bind the individual practitioner. HIPPA has clarified this issue: The act recognizes that agency personnel often work as teams, and it allows treatment teams to share protected health information as long as the client has been given the opportunity to object. Thus, clients should be informed that information is shared among treatment team members and that they can object to this. If they do object to information sharing, they must also be informed that staff may respond to their objection in whatever way seems most clinically appropriate, since HIPPA does not require that staff refrain from sharing information in the event of a patient objection.

As an example of the sort of problems that may emerge when prior consent is not obtained, consider the following: A therapist has been treating a 42-year-old woman with a personality disorder and he discovers that she has begun stealing office supplies and money from staff members' purses and wallets. When confronted with this discovery, she abruptly leaves treatment. Several months later, the therapist discovers that she has applied for treatment at another unit of the agency. He informs the staff there of her previous behavior, and she subsequently files an ethics charge, claiming breach of confidentiality. Although it is unlikely that severe ethical sanctions would result from this behavior, the difficulty could have been prevented by informing the woman of information-sharing practices when she began treatment.

Professional Needs (Consultation, Teaching, Support)

Certain threats to confidentiality emerge in the context of practitioners' relations with other professionals, particularly in consultation and teaching situations. In such roles, practitioners may want to use clinical information as examples or illustrations. The use of this information is not necessarily for the benefit of the client; rather, its purpose is to instruct. The ethical principles of various disciplines are ambiguous regarding these situations. They mandate either that the information be disguised so that the client is unidentifiable or that the client give consent before information is shared. The same guidance would apply to published case illustrations.

Practitioners also need support. For most, if not all, practitioners, the temptation to share clinical information with friends or family members can be overwhelming. At times, the practitioner may be feeling considerable stress and may need to ventilate or seek support. At other times, however, the motivation is simply to gossip or share an interesting story.

If the practitioner needs the support of a trusted and reliable intimate, he or she should obviously not reveal the identity of any client being discussed. In addition, the practitioner should also ensure that the confidant is aware and respectful of the highly sensitive and confidential nature of the information being shared. Such sharing should not be accomplished at the expense of the client's privacy or dignity. Discussions that fall into the latter category are those that serve primarily to entertain the audience, enhance the status of the speaker, or demean of subject of the story. These types of "sharing" would ordinarily be considered gossip.

Gossiping, especially gossiping that would threaten the client's dignity or make the practitioner appear unprofessional, should obviously be avoided. However, as Caruth (1985) has discussed, the motivation to gossip may stem from a need to create distance from the client. Additionally, professional gossip may serve as a means of competing with or establishing superiority over one's colleagues. Consider the following example: A clinician meets the supervisor (another mental health professional) of one of her clients at a party. In the context of a discussion of dissociative disorders, the clinician comments, "I'm working with one of your supervisees, and she's the worst borderline I've ever dealt with." The consequences of such a conversation should be obvious. Careless remarks made in settings where privacy is absent (e.g., cafeterias, parking lots, elevators), are similar ethical and professional lapses.

Managed Care Requirements

Of increasing concern are the threats to confidentiality arising out of the managed care environment. While clinicians have considerable ability to safeguard confidential information within their own walls, they lose this ability when information is provided to payors. With the influence of managed care agencies growing, the amount of information payors require is increasing, and often the information requested is clinical in nature. Because the trend has shifted from simply documenting diagnosis and number of sessions to a very specific analysis of each client, their problems, and the nature and duration of by the practitioner, there is no practical way that he or she can limit its use or dissemination once it is validly released by the patient. Horror stories abound regarding egregious breaches of confidentiality (J. R. Davidson & T. Davidson, 1996).

The clinician's ethical role in such situations is unclear. It may be argued that the practitioner has no ethical obligation to safeguard this information once it is released to the third-party payor on the basis of appropriate informed consent. In fact, there is little that the clinician can practically do, as is reflected in the fact that no codes of ethics specify the clinician's responsibility to safeguard records that have been duly released to third-party payors. On the other hand, it seems cavalier simply to say that protecting confidentiality is "not our job" in such cases.

While we await further guidelines on the protection of information once it is released to managed care entities, there are a few specific steps we can suggest:

1. Be sure that the client's consent is truly "informed" and that he or she knows how the information will be used and who will have access to it.
2. As noted in Chapter 10, chart entries should not contain extraneous information. One way to protect information in records is not to enter superfluous or unnecessarily detailed information in the first place.
3. The clinician should keep abreast of current legal and judicial efforts at protecting the confidentiality of medical records. Standards are evolving continually, particularly on the federal level.

    Practitioners should keep abreast of federal statutes that may affect their confidentiality practices, such as the Health Insurance Portability and Accountability Act.

GUIDELINES: WHEN TO BREACH CONFIDENTIALITY

In the course of clinical practice, a professional is certain to face numerous situations in which he or she will have to consider breaching confidentiality. For example, a child reveals that she has been sexually abused, a client shows signs of being suicidal or violent, or a request for information is received from a referring practitioner or family member. In some cases, the appropriate decision may be clear-cut, but others may place significant demands on the clinician's judgment.

Based on the preceding considerations and using the key questions from the flow chart presented in Chapter 2, some guidelines can be generated from its components regarding when it may be appropriate to breach confidentiality:

1. *Does a relevant, professional, legal, or social standard exist?* In this case, the relevant standard is that information obtained in the course of treatment is confidential unless the law mandates otherwise.
2. *Is there a reason to deviate from the standard?* Keeping in mind that confidentiality is a means to an end and that per-

fect confidentiality is practically impossible to guarantee, is there another ethical principle or legal requirement that justifies breaching confidentiality? A request for information from a family member, for instance, may not satisfy this requirement unless competing ethical or legal principles such as welfare of the client are raised. However, the duty to protect or report may constitute such a reason to deviate.

An important facet of dealing with this question is whether a solution that does not require breaching confidentiality can be generated. For instance, a practitioner may be satisfied that a potentially suicidal patient's "no-suicide contract" will be adhered to, may have an excellent therapeutic relationship with the patient, and may have ensured that the preferred means of self-destruction (e.g., pills, knife, gun) have been removed; in such a case, he or she may be able to avoid the need to contact family members and breach confidentiality.

3. *Can a primary ethical dimension be specified?* In some cases, only one ethical dimension will be obvious, but frequently such cases present little difficulty, at least from the perspective of determining which course of action is ethically appropriate (*implementing* the appropriate action, of course, may be extremely complicated—see below). In the majority of cases in which there are ethical dilemmas, more than one ethical issue may be at stake. Although deciding which ethical dimension is "primary" can be quite subjective, there are certainly occasions when such a determination can be made. Decision making can be simplified in such cases by focusing on the most important ethical issue.

4. *Does the new course of action appear to satisfy the needs/preferences of affected parties?* The principle of autonomy (as well as the aims of much mental health work) suggests that including the wishes of affected parties or "stakeholders" is an important component of ethically appropriate and nonpaternalistic action. While it is not always possible to obtain information about the "real" needs or preferences of stakeholders, educated guesses can be made, consultation can be

obtained, and a determination made as to whether the considered action is likely to satisfy affected parties.

5. *Does the course of action present any new ethical problems?* The practitioner should be deliberate in determining this course of action so that confidentiality is breached to the smallest extent necessary to accomplish the required task. For example, if the police need to be notified about a potentially violent act, they do not need to be told other details about treatment. The act of breaching confidentiality can only be justified if a greater good is accomplished by doing so.

6. *Can the course of action be implemented?* The question of practicality is always a consideration. For instance, if a potentially violent client does not meet the legal requirements for commitment, then commitment is obviously not a practical alternative, and there is no reason to breach confidentiality to get a client committed.

Chapter 5

INFORMED CONSENT

Providing the prospective client with the opportunity to give informed consent, implicitly or explicitly, forms a substantial portion of the concerns expressed in the various mental health professions' codes of ethics. However, the reason for this intense focus may not be immediately apparent. What is wrong with, for example, the traditional standard of "doctor knows best"? According to this standard, the patient simply presents himself or herself for treatment, and the doctor tells the patient what to do in order to effect a cure. This approach rests largely on the ethical principle of *beneficence,* which holds that to do good is the ultimate good.

This approach has several shortcomings, however. First, and perhaps most important from an analysis of ethical principles, the "doctor knows best" standard restricts the *autonomy* of the individual. The principle of autonomy holds that it is an ultimate value to treat individuals as free agents. For a professional to act in such a way as to restrict patients' autonomy deprives them of a crucial aspect of their humanness; it may also carry the implication that patients are incapable of making intelligent decisions about their treatment. The obligation to obtain patients' informed consent thus implies a respect for their dignity that rests on fundamental moral assumptions about the nature of the person.

Second, the "doctor knows best" standard is, unfortunately, too easy to abuse. In a number of highly publicized incidents (primarily in medicine) a patient or clinical research subject was damaged by treatment (or failure to give an indicated treatment) as a direct result of the provider's or researcher's failure to inform (cf. Faden et al., 1986). Although rare, such incidents occur in psychotherapy as well (cf. *Abraham v. Zaslow,* 1970/1974).

Third, the "doctor knows best" standard restricts the chances for the patient to actively participate in his or her own treatment. Especially in mental health work, this is a vital part of successful intervention. The passive patient is perhaps more tolerable in conventional medicine (although evidence is beginning to contradict this long-held belief), but in the psychological domain, simply to tell the patient "sit there and take your medicine" is either nonsensical or actually closes off a potent avenue of healing.

Thus, the obligation to inform the patient sufficiently that he or she can make a reasoned judgment about accepting or rejecting the proposed treatment is a significant one for the ethical mental health practitioner. It is also a procedure of prudence. Specifically, the therapeutic relationship, and, in fact, any voluntary professional relationship, rests on the consent of the client who initiated it. Moreover, the patient alone has the authority to terminate the relationship without censure. If professionals terminate a treatment relationship without the patient's consent for reasons of their own convenience, they are open to charges of abandonment. Clients have no such obligations and may unilaterally terminate a professional relationship unless they have been legally committed to treatment.

Despite the clear-cut obligation to inform prospective consumers so that they may make informed decisions, the specifics of providing opportunities for informed consent are far from clear. In part, this is a result of the fact that providing informed consent is both a moral obligation and an exercise of technical skill which will vary depending on the specifics of the case at hand. That is, the manner in which the practitioner provides information and the timing with which he or she provides it can affect whether the information is helpful or harmful. This will be discussed further below.

One often-overlooked benefit of this emphasis on informed consent is that obtaining it may enhance the trust between patient and provider. This issue is effectively discussed, primarily with regard to medicine, by Jonsen et al. (1998). These authors also note that there is yet another practical reason for obtaining informed consent: increasingly the courts recognize failure to obtain it as evidence of professional negligence.

The idea that one can obtain informed consent from prospective patients implies that they are able to absorb and process information so that they can voluntarily decide whether to utilize mental health services. It is true that some clinicians do not consider prospective mental health patients to be capable of autonomous action because of their psychological disturbance (Faden et al., 1986). However, because any given prospective patient's degree of disturbance is unknown when treatment is begun, the individual should be treated as if he or she has the capacity to act autonomously until there is evidence to the contrary. One simple way to articulate this standard is that the responsible mental health practitioner should attempt to obtain the maximum possible informed consent from patients or clients. Granted, this will not solve all dilemmas (e.g., consider the refusal of a severely mentally ill homeless person to accept referral to a facility), but it is a useful starting point.

This chapter discusses the nature of informed consent from a legal and a psychological perspective; it then discusses the necessary ingredients of informed consent; and finally, it addresses the limitations or exceptions to the obligation to provide informed consent.

THE NATURE OF INFORMED CONSENT

Three components are generally considered critical in obtaining informed consent. First, the idea that consent is *informed* implies that enough information has been provided for the potential client to make a reasonable determination whether to accept the recommended treatment. Second, the implicit notion underlying informed consent is that it is *voluntary.* Third, the implication in the notion of informed consent is that the consenter is *competent* to make such a determination. Competency refers to the ability to initiate a voluntary action and determine one's choices with at least the degree of autonomy possessed by the average member of one's culture or society.

A corollary of the preceding is that the provider must give information in such a manner that the prospective consumer can understand it. This means that the practitioner should avoid mystifying jargon and should use language comprehensible to the prospective client.

What are the standards for providing such information? One often-used standard has been the "usual and customary professional" standard. That is, the clinician is obligated to tell patients only that which the typical provider in his or her community tells patients. This standard has increasingly given way to the "reasonable person" standard, under which the provider must inform the client of any information that might be expected to affect a reasonable person's decision about the recommended procedure. There is, additionally, the less widely used standard called the "subjective understanding" standard (Faden et al., 1986). This standard indicates that the practitioner should provide any information that would be material and relevant to the *particular person* to whom the information is being disclosed. This standard, as Faden et al. discuss, is more difficult to implement in actual practice since it requires that the practitioner know a considerable amount about the prospective patient before treatment begins.

Information that is often desired by "reasonable persons" includes the likely duration of treatment, the fact that treatment is voluntary, and the general obligations one expects from patients (e.g., how much notice to give on cancelling appointments, permissibility of home telephone calls, charges for telephone consultations and report writing, if any). In addition, it is appropriate to offer information about the qualifications of the provider.

In determining what to include as part of an informed consent statement, the practitioner also must be cautious about information that may create a self-fulfilling prophecy. For instance, to inform a client that some people find psychotherapy stigmatizing may induce the client to respond to people in a more reserved or suspicious manner and, thus, affect the way the client is responded to by others.

By the same token, it could be argued that providing information about positive benefits that the treatment has produced will motivate clients' participation. The line between discussing the benefits of treatment and guaranteeing a particular outcome should be noted. Inclusion of a specific projected outcome in an informed consent statement could be viewed as a contractual obligation and increase the liability risk of the practitioner (Kenneth Pope, personal communication, 1983). On the other hand, the work of

Kahneman and Tversky (1981, 1984) suggests that informing clients about the *benefits* to be obtained from the proposed procedures often is superior to providing the same information couched in "harms to be avoided" when eliciting their consent. Faden et al. (1986) discuss this issue further; we mention it here to alert the practitioner to consider that the same information can be presented or framed in more than one way.

TAILORING DISCLOSURE TO THE SPECIFIC PERSON

The reality of providing information to patients so that they may make informed decisions is relatively complex. A few examples will illustrate the problem. When one asks what information will be relevant to which consumer with which problem, the actual consent disclosure becomes much more problematic. Does the single retiree who is presenting with problems of depression want to know that you are obligated to report him if he abuses his child (which he doesn't have)? Does the acutely psychotic patient want to know that one of the risks of therapy is that other people may find it a sign of poor adjustment? Clearly, certain information is not relevant to certain individuals. On the other hand, it may be highly relevant to inform a prospective client that his or her insurance company will be asking for information about the diagnosis before deciding whether to reimburse. Thus, it is often difficult to determine in advance what information will be needed by a particular client. On balance, it is probably better to give too much information than too little.

Tactics of Obtaining Informed Consent

There is both a content dimension to the task of obtaining informed consent and a process dimension. The content consists of essential information needed by prospective clients in order to enable them to make an informed decision. We present what we consider to be the seven minimum domains of information below:

1. *The Risks and Benefits of Treatment.* Depending on the setting in which one practices, risks could include the embarrassment of having other people know that one is receiving mental health treatment, the stirring up of unpleasant memories, the concern that others may think one

is mentally unstable, and difficulties of obtaining later employment (particularly relevant to accepting inpatient treatment). The benefits of treatment typically include more effective functioning in social, work, and family settings; decreased negative emotionality; less self-defeating behavior; improved ability to realize life goals; and more satisfying relationships.

2. *Logistics of Treatment.* Typically this information might include how long sessions last (e.g., 50-minute "hours"), how long treatment lasts (e.g., weekly for several months, twice-weekly for several years, etc.), the cost of sessions, the cost of additional services such as telephone contact, letter writing on behalf of the client, testing and test interpretation, types of records kept, billing practices, and policies regarding insurance reimbursement.

3. *Qualifications of the Provider.* Ordinarily this includes highest degree obtained; provider's specialty (e.g., psychology, social work, psychiatry, marriage and family therapy, counseling); board certifications, if any; additional specialty, if any (e.g., hypnosis, family therapy, gestalt, biofeedback); particular disorders or issues emphasized in practice (e.g., divorce, sexual dysfunction, substance abuse); and training and experience in the kind of service being sought by this client (if not covered in the previous items).

4. *Risks and Benefits of Alternatives to Treatment.* In addition to describing what treatment might help to accomplish and what risks it might entail, it may be important to provide parallel information regarding the alternatives to treatment. If there are well-accepted alternatives to the type of treatment one offers, these should be mentioned to the prospective client. If the only alternative to the treatment one offers is no treatment, then the risks of allowing the condition to remain untreated should be explained. Typically, these risks include risk that the condition will simply persist if left untreated, risk that the condition will worsen, and risk that it will become less amenable to treatment over time.

An interesting derivative question is whether the provider is obligated to disclose the risks and benefits of treatments of which he or she disapproves (cf. Jonsen et al., 1998). From an ethical point of view, the practitioner is *permitted* but not *obligated* to disclose such information. However, from a technical or clinical point of view, the practitioner may prefer to disclose such information as a means of more strongly recommending the treatment of choice.

5. *Clarity Regarding Technique.* In the past it was common to remind therapists to obtain informed consent about any "unusual" methods they employed or unusual policies they followed. However, because treatment is so variable across settings and across providers, the definition of "unusual" depends heavily on one's viewpoint. Therefore, therapists should provide as much clarity as they think is necessary regarding their techniques. For example, some therapists use homework assignments, some use concurrent group therapy, some require certain tests, some routinely schedule family sessions, and some routinely make tape recordings of sessions.

6. *Emergency Procedures.* The therapist should have a backup or emergency service, and these arrangements should be described. If there is no such service and the therapist has particular recommendations for clients who need after-hours contact, these policies should be described. For example, does the therapist take "crisis" calls at home after hours? Alternatively, does the therapist not publish his or her phone number and instead refer clients to the local crisis line of the community mental health center? What information, if any, is provided to covering therapists in the clinician's absence?

7. *Confidentiality and Its Limits.* Although it is commonly expected by prospective clients that confidentiality will be upheld (McGuire, Toal, & Blau, 1985; Rubanowitz, 1987), it is helpful to remind clients both that the information they provide will be held confidential and that there are certain limits to this protection. As noted earlier, it is not technically required that therapists inform their clients about the possibility that they will be obliged to breach confidentiality in cases of potential harm to self or others; however, it is wise to mention the "duty to protect" issue at the outset. Including this information reduces the chance that the client will accuse the therapist of entrapment after the

client has revealed information that signals dangerousness. Similar suggestions can be made regarding reporting
laws for cases of child abuse, incest, spouse abuse, the
planning of crimes, and suicide risk (Crenshaw &
Lichtenberg, 1993).

How to Include Information

Because many patients are eager to "get on" with the discussion of their chief complaint, some practitioners have raised the
question of whether it unnecessarily delays treatment (and would
therefore be ethically undesirable) to provide the necessary information about treatment and obtain informed consent at the outset.
In an interesting ethics case involving a mental health professional
who failed to disclose his fees to a client, the defense to the lapse
by the clinician was that "therapy had not really begun" since this
particular therapist considered the first three to five sessions to be
"evaluation" and not "treatment." Needless to say, the client (now
ex-client and complainant) prevailed and the therapist was disciplined.

With the most recent revisions of the major mental health
professions' ethics codes, this issue of timing is now moot; all
specify professionals' obligations to inform users of their services
(and any other relevant information) at the outset of treatment.
The psychologists' ethics code (American Psychological Association, 2002) mandates that "psychologists inform clients/patients
as early as is feasible in the therapeutic relationship about the nature and anticipated course of therapy, fees, involvement in third
parties, and limits of confidentiality" (§ 10.01a). The psychiatrists'
code of ethics (American Psychiatric Association, 2001) indicates
that "Psychiatric services, like all medical services, are dispensed
in the context of a contractual arrangement between the patient
and the physician. The provisions of the contractual arrangement,
which are binding on the physician as well as on the patient, should
be explicitly established" (§ 2.5). Social workers "should provide
information about the nature and extent of services and about the
extent of clients' right to refuse service" (NASW, 1999, § 1.03d).
The marriage and family therapists' code (AAMFT, 2001) states,
"Marriage and family therapists obtain appropriate informed consent to therapy or related procedures as early as feasible in the

therapeutic relationship, and use language that is reasonably understandable to clients" (§ 1.2). Counselors "inform clients of the purposes, goals, techniques, procedures, limitations, potential risks, and benefits of services to be performed, and other pertinent information" (ACA, 1995, A.3.a).

Nonetheless, despite the need for full disclosure and informed consent, there is an element of beneficence in the wish to delay treatment of a distressed individual as little as possible. One possible resolution to the problem is to provide written informed consent statements.

Written Informed Consent

Written informed consent statements or "patient information" statements allow some of the treatment issues to be presented and digested before the session begins. Less pressing questions can be dealt with later. This approach too has its advantages and drawbacks. As an advantage, it saves the practitioner the time needed to detail the many possible risks and benefits of treatment, and it also removes some of the more difficult issues from immediate presentation. As a disadvantage, it does not allow the practitioner to assess carefully whether the patient indeed comprehends the proposed treatment. Written promises are also frequently treated as evidence of contractual liability, so such statements must be prepared with extra care (this may be an advantage). A written patient information statement is rapidly becoming the standard of practice (Bennett et al., 1990). Although Bennett et al. do not specifically recommend written informed consent statements, they do recommend that if written statements are *not* used, that documentation of the clinician's obtaining informed consent be included in the record. A sample disclosure form developed and used by one of the authors (LJH) in a general outpatient psychology practice is included with the present volume as Appendix F (pp. 319-320). The example statement includes the "minimum elements" of informed consent and treatment contract documents (Kennedy et al., 2003). It is offered in the hope that others may use and improve upon it; in the interests of fully informing the reader of the risks and benefits, it should be clear that the responsibility for adapting the statement to one's own state laws, practice environment, and patient population is entirely the user's. Additional examples of patient information and/or treatment contract forms can be found in Bennett et al. (1990).

Written information statements have several advantages: The information can be presented comprehensively, it can be written clearly (editorial consultation may be helpful in this area), and it allows the client to absorb the information at his or her own rate. In addition, written information is consistent across clients and can be given to patients at the beginning of therapy without interfering unduly with the establishment of the working relationship. Further, written informed consent statements leave a record that one has at least offered certain facts for the client's consideration (whether the client absorbs those facts is another story). Finally the provision of an informed consent statement can serve in part to establish an atmosphere of openness about one's services. Of course, it is also possible to send the message that one is legalistically defensive about one's practice. However, with consultation from knowledgeable colleagues and possibly even provisional documents offered to clients for their feedback, the written informed consent statement can be refined to send the message that one is willing to be clear with clients about their rights.

Verbal Informed Consent

Informed consent should also be obtained verbally. Verbal informed consent allows the careful assessment of the individual's comprehension of the issues, allows for the providing of information specific to the client's circumstances, and permits the communication of positive affect (such as caring, consideration, kindness, affirmation of the client's independence, respect) that the written format does not permit.

Verbal informed consent can be obtained both "proactively" and "reactively." By proactively obtaining verbal informed consent it is meant that providers should, some time after giving the written document to clients, check to see if the material has been read and understood. The written document may trigger questions which the therapist can then answer. Reactively obtaining verbal informed consent means that the therapist assumes that the client will ask questions if he or she is unclear about an aspect of treatment and is ready to respond to such questions. The nature of the questions triggered by various events in therapy cannot be predicted, but they usually touch on issues that should have already been presented in the early phases. Of course, one must first establish a climate in which clients feel free to ask such questions. It is remarkable how often clients feel intimidated by their therapists and do not feel free to ask (cf. Dimatteo & Hendricks, 1982).

The Informed Consent Attitude

Informed consent can be obtained in either a defensive, legalistic manner or in an open, trust-building way. Much of this contextual information is sent nonverbally, and much of it depends on the therapist's own level of comfort with his or her practices. The informed consent procedure can be considered as a specific example of a person-environment interaction; the therapist has several parts to play in establishing the appropriate environment: First and foremost, the therapist must be fair with the client without being discouraging about the realities of treatment outcome. On the other hand, the clinician must be optimistic and validate the client's faith in the process without overselling the treatment. No hard-and-fast rules are possible in this regard. A judgment about the client's level of optimism/pessimism, one's own mastery or lack of mastery of the techniques, and the difficulty of the problem at hand all contribute to a contextual judgment of what to say and how to say it. Nonetheless it is hard to imagine "losing therapeutic ground" by treating clients as if they are potential collaborators in their own treatment. Indeed, that is the ultimate goal of much psychotherapy. Informed consent increases the likelihood that clients can challenge what their therapists offer them, and this in turn makes it important to be comfortable with what one does. Indeed, the question of the boundary between appropriate curiosity about aspects of treatment and resistance to such treatment is always a clinical issue to be resolved. Therapists, too, need to resolve the question of when they are simply being withholding because they feel restricted in their practice and when they are intuitively picking up some defensive purpose to the repeated questions raised by clients.

The conventional view of informed consent procedures suggests that all issues be spelled out at the beginning of treatment; however, this may be clinically unrealistic because it would leave little time for actual clinical work if carried to its logical extreme. Thus it may be more useful to consider the obtaining of informed consent as a process, perhaps beginning with more general and global descriptions of the elements of treatment and later progressing to specific descriptions of specific procedures as needed.

LIMITATIONS TO INFORMED CONSENT

Although the paradigm for providing information to prospective consumers is that the consumer is an independent, autonomous, competent adult, in reality many other conditions apply. These conditions can compromise any of the aforementioned characteristics. For example, the person may not be considered competent by reason of disabling mental status or of youth, the person may not be in the position to make an informed judgment because of the time pressures or emergency nature of the situation, the person may not be able to consent because of legal constraints, or consent may be limited because of judgment by the professional that the risks of harming the patient through disclosure outweigh the benefits to be gained by involving the patient in a participatory decision. Each of these will be considered in turn below.

Youth

The legal age for competence to consent (to such things as contracts and marriages as well as mental health treatment) varies somewhat from state to state and situation to situation but is typically around age 16 (Jacob & Hartshorne, 2003; Plotkin, 1981). This age marker is simply a "proxy" for other characteristics that are assumed to change with age. These include the ability to weigh the consequences of a present course of action for one's future well-being. In the obvious case—that is, a child who is clearly unable to understand the nature of treatment but who obviously needs it—one finds "substituted consent." That is, the responsible party, usually a parent or guardian, consents for the minor. Many authors (e.g., Schetky & Cavanaugh, 1982) note that either parent's consent suffices when the parents are married. However, when divorce has occurred, clinicians must ascertain who has legal custody and obtain consent from that parent. In cases of joint custody, it is prudent to obtain consent from both parents. If legal guardianship resides elsewhere, that person or agency must give consent.

From a clinical standpoint, it is wise to attempt to maximize the child's understanding of the proposed treatment. This is known as obtaining minors' *assent* (Jacob & Hartshorne, 2003). As these authors and others (e.g., Holder, 1985; Melton, 1981) point out, involving children in treatment decisions improves treatment outcome. Weithorn (1983) cites several studies that have shown, in addition, that the process of involving a child in health-related decision making contributes to an increased sense of personal responsibility for health care. However, from an ethical point of view, involving the child is aspirational rather than mandatory, and from a legal point of view it is usually superfluous. The converse— failure to obtain parental permission—may engender legal and practical, as well as ethical, problems, however. As Schetkey and Cavanaugh (1982) point out, such failure can expose the practitioner to a legal risk of assault (unwanted "touching") if challenged by an aggrieved parent, and may also result in disputes over payment of the bill. As the child enters middle to late adolescence, however, the issue becomes more confusing.

Gaylin (1982) has usefully discriminated between the child's ability to independently *consent* to treatment versus the child's ability to independently *refuse* treatment. Gaylin suggests that the practitioner should give greater weight to the child's willingness to accept treatment in the face of parental disapproval and somewhat less weight to the child's ability to independently refuse treatment in the face of parental interest in continuing or initiating it. When professionals examine these concepts, it becomes clear that one underlying dimension is the question of the person's judgments about short-term benefits versus long-term costs and benefits. This analysis of the situation suggests that the youngster who is willing to undergo short-term "costs" (e.g., treatment) in the interest of long-term benefits should be taken seriously; however, if the youngster seems to prefer short-term "benefits" (e.g., avoidance of treatment) regardless of long-term "costs" of such a course of action, perhaps more effort should be made to recruit him or her into treatment.

Diminished Capacity

In the case of psychotic, retarded, or demented individuals who lack the capacity to give competent informed consent, the concept of "substituted consent" can supplement or replace issues of obtaining informed consent from the patient himself or herself. When it is clear that an individual does not have the capacity to rationally weigh the costs and benefits of treatment, a third party who may be assumed to have the patient's interests at stake can be consulted. It may be the case that no such third party exists, and in such cases the practitioner should turn to an informed party of peers or laypersons. Even in cases of substituted consent, however, it is useful to at least provide the individual an opportunity to assent to the proposed treatment.

Emergencies

True life-threatening emergencies in mental health practice are fortunately rather rare. Typically it is possible to provide the prospective patient with at least a brief description of what is proposed without unduly delaying treatment or causing damage. This is in contrast to the medical situation, in which delay of even a few minutes may be dangerous or in which the patient may present in an unconscious state. Nonetheless it occasionally does occur that patients present with acute mental health emergencies. What are such emergencies? A primary one concerns the suicidal patient. Such individuals are in need of immediate psychological intervention, and clinicians are probably more concerned about their continued survival than informing them about the long-term costs and benefits of entering treatment.

A second situation that makes it difficult to provide informed consent is that in which a psychotic episode is occurring. Individuals in psychotic states cannot usually be considered competent to provide informed consent. Thus if the situation is one in which time makes a difference, treatment may reasonably be started without obtaining informed consent. If there is more time available, patients' guardians, relatives, or "substituted consent providers" should be contacted. In such cases it is usually permissible to use one's professional judgment to initiate treatment and to delay providing information relevant to informed consent until such time as it may be useful to the patient. Notice that once again the principles of autonomy and beneficence are in conflict, with beneficence winning out.

Legal Constraints

In certain cases the patient's participation in treatment is nonvoluntary. Such cases include court-ordered treatment (in which case it might reasonably be argued that the "patient" is the court, at least as much as is the individual sitting in the consulting room).

Other such cases include those in which a spouse has threatened consequences such as divorce if the person does not seek treatment. These cases are somewhat more difficult if they raise questions about the voluntariness of the consent obtained. As in the preceding case, this raises the question "Who is the client?" Particularly in cases in which the identified client appears to be feeling coerced, the clinician must carefully evaluate whether the party insisting on treatment should be included in the negotiation of the treatment contract. This may prevent later difficulties if the insistent party is dissatisfied with the progress of therapy. However, even in the absence of clear indications of coercion, the therapist should be especially sensitive to the client's treatment options. If the client cannot be voluntarily involved in the choice of treatment directions (even if he or she might not have chosen to be in treatment), then termination should be considered. The ethical codes of almost all the mental health professions mandate terminating a nonproductive professional relationship, and this policy is consistent with such a mandate.

Professional Judgment

Practitioners should use their professional judgment when it appears that providing informed consent will damage the patient in some way, or in cases in which there is some theoretical rationale for withholding information. It is useful to remember that the provision of informed consent is a means to an end. It is not an end in itself. The end is to emphasize the autonomy and dignity of the individual. This can be done through other means if providing informed consent would potentially harm the treatment relationship or drive the person from suitable treatment. These kinds of cases invoke the conflicting principle of beneficence in contrast to the principle of autonomy.

Hypnotic techniques, especially in Ericksonian therapy, bear on this issue, as do some attempts to enhance transference. Paradoxical therapy (defined by Rohrbaugh [1982] as instructing the client to intensify or enact situations that were described by the client as undesirable) is also problematic. The therapist is directing the client to do something which the therapist does not actually believe the client should do. Examples of paradoxical suggestions include indicating to clients that they "become more depressed" or suggesting that clients intensify a particular symptom at a particular time. Should the therapist inform the client that actually the therapist is giving these instructions so that the client can get rid of the symptom in question? Many paradoxical therapists argue that revealing the fact that an instruction is intended to be paradoxical renders it useless.

For example, it is not uncommon for therapists who give "symptom prescriptions" as between-session assignments to be asked for the rationale behind this. Answering, "If you don't do this, I'll be forced to refer you" without any additional explanation is unnecessarily harsh (although actually recommended by some advocates). Instead, the therapist could indicate that in his or her best judgment, this technique may prove helpful and ask the client to try it as an "experiment." It should be noted in passing that there is no empirical support for the idea that informing patients about paradoxical methods reduces their effectiveness. For example, Hills, Gruszkos, and Strong (1985), found that outcomes for clients who were and were not informed about paradoxical techniques did not differ after 30 days. Similarly, Hunsley (1988) argues that providing a rationale does not reduce the usefulness of paradox any more than a rationale for any other intervention reduces its usefulness. Other studies (e.g., Ascher & Turner, 1980) also confirm the notion that paradox "works" even if it is explained. Thus there would appear to be little justification for failing to inform clients that one's directives and suggestions are, even if they appear contrary, designed to improve the client's well-being.

Psychotherapists who use psychoanalytic methods also seem to have trouble reconciling these principles. Such therapists argue that revealing too much about the technique to the patient can contribute to resistance and can interfere with effective treatment.

However, at the minimum it is clear that providing information is not a dichotomous task: One can certainly provide much essential information without going into technical detail about the nature of one's procedures. It certainly seems reasonable to inform patients that (a) treatment is voluntary, (b) techniques which may not always be of obvious relevance will be employed, and (c) they have the right to ask questions at any time. It seems to us that these concepts could be presented to clients without unduly compromising the therapist's effectiveness.

Summary: Guidelines for Providing Informed Consent

The following are practical guidelines for providing the opportunity for informed consent:

1. Assume that the person is competent to give informed consent unless there is clear evidence to the contrary.
2. Put yourself in the patient's place; what information would *you* desire?
3. Use clinical judgment in providing the details of the proposed treatment; how much information can the person absorb? Consider that information overload can prevent the obtaining of informed consent perhaps as much as underdisclosure.
4. If in doubt, inform the person anyway. It is always better to have informed than to be accused later of having denied the patient the opportunity to decide for himself or herself.
5. Put the standard treatment information in writing, give the client a copy of the statement (and keep a signed copy), and have respected colleagues review your statement.

Chapter 6

DUAL RELATIONSHIPS: AVOIDING EXPLOITATION AND MAINTAINING APPROPRIATE BOUNDARIES

Mental health practitioners occupy many roles in addition to those of psychotherapist, consultant, or evaluator. Such roles include neighbor, friend, relative, employer, or voter. Typically these roles do not conflict. But increasingly, as the size of the community in which one practices decreases or as the group with which one practices overlaps more and more with one's other social groups, practitioners run the risk of having additional role relationships with their patients or clients. Many of these "dual relationships" do not raise ethical questions. For example, one's client may also be one's neighbor and one may encounter this person at neighborhood association meetings or while working in one's yard. Aside from some possible momentary embarrassment and fleeting questions about how best to manage the interaction, this sort of dual relationship is not necessarily ethically problematic. Other dual relationships are more difficult. From an ethical and perhaps a technical standpoint as well, the roles of therapist and lover, therapist and employee, therapist and relative, therapist and instructor, or therapist and supervisor are not compatible. This chapter focuses on the range of dual relationships and offers some guidelines for maintaining one's ethical equilibrium.

Example 1. A male therapist is working with a female client. He has begun a practice of walking her to her car after their evening sessions, ostensibly to make sure she's safe. Then he begins scheduling her as his last client of the evening. One night, he asks her to have a drink with him, telling her that it would be therapeutic for her to associate with a decent man, as opposed to the losers with whom she usually spends her time. The client is flattered by all of the attention being showered upon her by a man for whom she has great respect, and she goes along with him. One thing leads to another, until eventually they end up in bed. The therapist tells her that sex with him would be good for her psychologically because he is the type of man she should be associating with; again, she is unquestioning in her trust of the therapist. As the relationships progress, the client begins writing the therapist love letters and calling him at home, and the frequency of such contacts increases to a point where the therapist's wife begins to ask questions. Finally, the therapist tells the client that she is not amenable to treatment and that she'll never change, and he abruptly terminates her (from both relationships).

Example 2. A therapist is the coach of her 10-year-old daughter's volleyball team. One of the girls on the team is having a terrible time controlling her anxiety, and her performance during games deteriorates because she is so tense. The therapist discusses the problem with the girl's parents and suggests that they make an appointment to bring the girl in for desensitization therapy. Unfortunately, the girl's anxiety does not improve with treatment, and in fact she gets worse. She tells her parents that she dreads going to practice because she is afraid that she will disappoint her therapist/coach. Her attendance at practices and games becomes more and more sporadic, and she finally drops off the team.

Example 3. Over the course of therapy, a therapist who is treating a couple begins to develop a fondness for them, and they for him. The couple invites the therapist and his wife to a party, and his wife also develops a fondness for the couple. The two couples spend increasing amounts of time together, while the therapist continues to work with them. At a later party, the couple begins to quarrel and attempts to involve the therapist.

Though different in many ways, these examples represent several of the countless instances of problematic dual relationships that can develop. While the term "multiple relationships" has seen increased use in the past years and has become the term used in the *Ethical Principles of Psychologists and Code of Conduct* (American Psychological Association, 2002), we have opted to continue using the term "dual relationships" to describe this particular sort of ethical problem. While it is true that a practitioner and a consumer of services can be involved in more than two relationships, it is easier to assess the problematic nature of relationships and to evaluate the relevant ethical issues if they are considered two at a time (e.g., a therapist-client relationship combined with a romantic relationship or a consultant-consultee relationship combined with a financial relationship).

As noted previously, many dual relationships do not raise ethical questions, while others are more problematic. The affective and clinical aspects of dual relationships and boundary maintenance have been addressed in depth elsewhere (e.g., Glass, 2003; Norris, Gutheil, & Strasburger, 2003; Reamer, 2003) and from an exploited patient's personal perspective (Roy & Freeman, 1976). This chapter will discuss a number of practical and ethical aspects of dual relationships. We will first discuss general problems that arise when a therapist and a client maintain a dual relationship. Then, some aspects of dual relationships particularly relevant to clinical practice will be described. Finally, we will present guidelines for avoiding potentially problematic dual relationships and maintaining one's ethical equilibrium.

WHEN AND WHY ARE DUAL RELATIONSHIPS BAD?

Because we are all human beings it is impossible for us to avoid dual relationships completely. Dual relationships are made almost inevitable by the fact that we all exist in social worlds and interact with people in numerous contexts. The likelihood of encountering a client outside the therapeutic setting is substantial, and it increases with the years a professional has been in practice. In fact, some extratherapy relationships are a vital source of referrals, and it would raise other ethical questions to refuse to offer services to persons with whom one had other contacts.

The smaller the community, the greater are the chances that dual relationships will develop, until at some point they become a virtual certainty. For instance, a social worker of our acquaintance was asked to conduct family therapy with the family of his own brother—there were simply no other available family therapists (or other types of mental health professionals, for that matter) in the small town in which he practiced. Considerable attention has been paid to the special problems of dual relationships encountered in rural communities (Helbok, 2003; Jennings, 1992; Stockman, 1990). It is important to keep in mind that dual relationships are not inherently unethical. No code of ethical standards for the major mental health professions prohibits all dual relationships, but each stresses the obligation of the ethical professional to be aware of the potential harm that could be caused by dual relationships. There also seems to be an increased awareness that dual relationships cannot be avoided completely. For instance, the AAMFT *Code of Ethics* (2001) states, "Therapists, therefore, make every effort to avoid conditions and multiple relationships with clients that could impair professional judgment or increase the risk of exploitation. Such relationships include, but are not limited to, business or close personal relationships with a client or the clients' immediate family. When the risk of impairment or exploitation exists due to conditions or multiple roles, therapists take appropriate precautions" (§ 1.3).

The *Ethical Principles of Psychologists and Code of Conduct* (American Psychological Association, 2002) states, "A psychologist refrains from entering into a multiple relationship if the multiple relationship could reasonably be expected to impair the psychologist's objectivity, competence, or effectiveness in performing his or her functions as a psychologist, or otherwise risks exploitation or harm to the person with whom the professional relationship exists (Standard 3.05a). The *Code of Ethics and Standards of Practice* of the American Counseling Association (1995) makes a very similar statement (§ A.6.a).

According to the NASW *Code of Ethics* (NASW, 1999), "Social workers should not engage in dual or multiple relationships with clients or former clients in which there is a risk of exploitation or potential harm to the client. In instances when dual or multiple relationships are unavoidable, social workers should take steps to protect clients and are responsible for setting clear, appropriate, and culturally sensitive boundaries" (§ 1.06c). While not specifically using the term "dual relationships," *The Principles of Medical Ethics With Annotations Especially Applicable to Psychiatry* (American Psychiatric Association, 2001) raises related issues that are of ethical concern. For instance, it states, "The psychiatrist should diligently guard against exploiting information furnished by the patient and should not use the unique position of power afforded him/her by the psychotherapeutic situation to influence the patient in any way not directly relevant to the treatment goals" (§ 2.2).

The preceding statements highlight some of the potential problems that can occur if a therapist maintains a dual relationship with a client. Listed below are two specific concerns:

1. *Dual relationships may exploit the client.* The therapeutic relationship involves an asymmetry of power; the therapist discloses little and comes to know the person at his or her most vulnerable point. Because of this asymmetry, it is doubtful whether the client could distinguish between times when the therapist is acting as a therapist and when he or she is acting as a friend, colleague, or the like. There are real questions as to whether a client could make a truly autonomous decision in the face of persuasion by the therapist. If the therapist suggested, for instance, that the client participate in a business venture, would the client be able to distinguish the therapist as a good clinician from the therapist as a bad business person, and would the client be able to refuse without wondering whether the treatment upon which he or she had come to depend might be jeopardized?

2. *Dual relationships may affect the therapist's ability to make appropriate clinical decisions.* If a practitioner maintains a friendship or other nonclinical relationship with a client, this may make it difficult to confront that client about inappropriate behavior. It may also affect the type of recommendations that the clinician would make about the client. It may be hard, for example, to tell a client with

whom you maintain a social relationship that you can understand why his children wish to live with their mother (his ex-wife), or that you see no clinically justifiable reason that he should not have to serve a jail sentence for a crime he has committed.

When dual relationships are involved, it becomes significantly more difficult for a clinician to be certain about his or her motives, a judgment which is difficult under the best circumstances. Given the human ability to rationalize, it is extremely easy to mask the real reason that a particular step is being taken behind a motive that sounds clinically justifiable. The practitioner should always be sensitive to this potential.

In summary, dual relationships cannot be avoided completely and are not inherently unethical. However, they provide fertile ground for the development of problematic situations and, therefore, caution is in order. Certain dual relationships, such as those involving sex with a current client, are always unethical, however. In the section below, some dual relationship situations that present special problems for the clinician are discussed.

CLINICALLY RELEVANT DUAL RELATIONSHIPS

Although the number of potential dual relationships is quite large, a smaller set merits special attention and will be described separately. These include accepting friends or acquaintances as clients, becoming friends with clients, receiving gifts, and engaging in sexual relationships with current or former clients.

Accepting Friends or Acquaintances As Clients

If a therapist were to decide to avoid dual relationships completely, then he or she would refuse to accept anyone as a client with whom there had been any previous nonclinical contact of any sort and would even refuse to accept anyone with whom he or she shared common friends or anyone with whom social contact might be a potential in the future. Few independently practicing therapists, however, have such an unlimited referral pool (or such clairvoyance) that they could be so restrictive although adopting this stance would eliminate a number of potential problems.

Rather, many (if not most) clinicians who are not affiliated with agencies take considerable advantage of referrals made by friends, acquaintances, and other individuals known in social contexts. In accepting clients from these sources, special care must be taken to ensure the same autonomy of decision making that the individual would have if the referral were from another source. This is because of the kinds of social obligations unique to this type of referral.

Consider the following possible client reaction, "I think this therapist is incompetent, but Brad and Susan like him, so if I say anything, I'm offending my friends." Or "If I tell my therapist I don't want any more counseling, I'm going to feel uncomfortable seeing her at the party next week."

The therapist must also examine the limits that the dual relationship will place on his or her response alternatives. If the therapist knows, for instance, that confronting the client will make him or her angry and that the client will likely react by making negative statements about the therapist to mutual friends, there might be a temptation to "pull one's punches" in nontherapeutic ways.

While not specifically an ethical concern, the therapist might be wise also to consider what practical limitations will be placed on his or her own social life if an individual is accepted as a client. Therapists are sometimes vulnerable to "supermarket consultations" with intrusive patients in any case; such encounters with a neighbor-client-friend might be even more difficult to avoid and to terminate gracefully. Therapists' lives could eventually become quite constricted unless they were particularly good (or insensitive) in setting limits on such informal consultations.

Once dual relationships that pose obvious problems in maintaining objectivity and professional distance—such as those with family members, close friends, coworkers, and subordinates—have been eliminated from consideration, the therapist should ask himself or herself the following questions before accepting as a client an acquaintance, a friend of a friend, or someone whose status raises the potential for a social dual relationship:

1.   Will the dual relationship inhibit in some way the client's ability to make autonomous decisions? Can you anticipate any ways in which the client will feel that he or she cannot disagree with you because of outside demands of any sort?

2. Will the dual relationship restrict your response alternatives? Can you act in the ways necessary and say the things necessary for effective treatment as you would with any other client?

3. Where do your motivations fit in? Are you likely to find yourself playing to an imagined audience rather than doing what is clinically right? Are you motivated to establish a great reputation or to meet some rescue fantasy? Can you resist these temptations?

Since the temptation to accept a client in this type of context may be strong, it is important that the clinician honestly grapple with these considerations. Inherent in such deliberations is a tendency to rationalize, which should be acknowledged and examined, as well. Here, as elsewhere, consultation with knowledgeable and trustworthy colleagues is extremely helpful.

Friendships With Clients

Given the intimate nature of the therapeutic relationship and the amount of time a therapist spends with clients, it is not difficult to understand the temptation to develop friendships with clients and to want to socialize with them. While such a temptation is natural, in general, we believe that such friendships should be avoided. A therapist-client relationship is based on trust, intimacy, and self-disclosure. Typically, the information flow goes one way. That is, the client shares much more personal information than does the therapist. The therapist, in turn, assumes an expert role— as one who is capable of handling such information sensitively and who is able to help the client.

This type of role definition has several consequences. Because of the time-limited and unique nature of the therapeutic relationship, a client is likely to self-disclose more than he or she would in a social relationship. An ongoing social relationship with a therapist, or the potential of one, may inhibit the client's self-disclosure or honesty. Further, it is unlikely that the therapist could act freely as a therapist and as a friend simultaneously—one relationship or the other would have to suffer. Perhaps the therapeutic relationship would break down in favor of a more symmetrical friendship, or the asymmetry of the therapeutic relationship would characterize the friendship, or there may be elements of both.

While these contentions may be sensible to consider during the process of therapy, one may assert that once therapy is terminated, there should be nothing to stand in the way of a social relationship. In contrast, we believe that the process of therapy in most cases prevents a truly symmetrical social relationship from ever being able to develop. The fact that the friendship had its genesis in a therapeutic relationship will make it impossible to know what the nature of the friendship would have been otherwise, and the freedom of action of both participants is likely to be limited in subtle ways. There is a question as to whether the ex-client could ever see the therapist in an objective light. It appears likely instead that there would always be some degree of distortion in the ex-client's view of the therapist. Further, if a social relationship is allowed to follow therapy, it is likely to preclude the possibility of that person's ever coming back into therapy with that therapist.

For the preceding reasons, the wise clinician should take appropriate steps to prevent the development of a friendship with a client, either during therapy or afterwards. This does not necessarily mean a rigid avoidance of social contact, but rather an expanded awareness of the potential for trouble.

Gifts from Clients

There are a number of reasons that a client may give a therapist a gift (Drew, Stoeckle, & Billings, 1983; Hundert, 1998). At times, gift giving can be an honest and sincere expression of appreciation for the help a therapist has provided. At other times, however, a gift may be given for other, more problematic reasons, for example, as a bid for a more social relationship with the therapist or as a means of asking the therapist to "go easy" on the client. There are also times when a gift is given as an out-and-out bribe—for instance, to motivate the therapist to write a helpful disability or workers' compensation evaluation.

It is not unethical in all situations to accept a gift from a client. In fact, it would be inappropriate and countertherapeutic to refuse a gift in some situations. On the other hand, accepting a gift would be clearly unethical in other situations. The *Code of Ethics* of the AAMFT (2001) acknowledges that gifts are not inherently unethical by stating that "Marriage and family therapists do not give to or receive from clients (a) gifts of substantial value or

(b) gifts that impair the integrity or efficacy of the therapeutic relationship" (§ 3.10).

A number of factors should be considered in deciding whether to accept a gift from a client:

1. What are the client's apparent motives for giving the gift? Does there seem to be any ulterior motive, either overt or covert, that applies? For instance, does the client need something from the therapist, such as a positive letter to a court, or does the client want to control the type of feedback he or she hears from the therapist?

2. Will the gift have an effect on treatment? While it is tempting to contend that the gift will have no impact on what the clinician says or does, a more honest analysis of feelings may reveal otherwise.

3. What is the value of the gift? It is easier to justify accepting a gift of little financial value than one of greater worth. Not only is the absolute cost of the gift relevant, but also the proportion of the client's income that the gift represents. A gift worth $25 may represent a significant proportion of the income of a single mother living on welfare, but perhaps only a token when given by a wealthy person. Don't overlook the symbolic value of the gift (Hundert, 1998).

4. What about the temporal context? A gift given during the holiday season or at the end of therapy may have a different meaning than one given at another time, or one accompanied by a statement such as, "I just saw this and it reminded me of you."

At times, a therapist may feel uncomfortable about accepting a gift but may not know how to refuse it or give it back without hurting the client or being countertherapeutic. Following are some suggestions on how to refuse a gift without being unduly rejecting or causing undue embarrassment to the client.

1. Express a positive, caring sentiment to the client, such as "I'm flattered by this, and pleased that you would feel so positive about your counseling experience, but I can't accept your generosity." ("Why not?" will be the response.)

2. Take responsibility for not being able to accept the gift, such as, "I know that you are giving me this in a positive, generous spirit, and I appreciate that, but in my experience therapy will go better if gifts aren't involved in our work."
3. Be deliberate and sensitive about how you clinically process the gift giving. While you may want to tuck it away and bring it up thematically later, a client is likely to feel hurt and rejected if your first response is, "This seems to be one more way in which you try to buy acceptance." It is also worth considering that a clinically significant theme will likely emerge more than once.
4. Suggest an alternative that allows the client to express gratitude without the therapist benefiting directly, for example, "Since I can't accept this piano, if you sincerely want to express your gratitude about the help you've gotten, you may want to donate it to the Children's Hospital." However, be cautious not to suggest that the patient should be donating in your name to the charity of your choice.
5. Be relaxed. If the clinician conveys a sense of discomfort and uncertainty about how to handle the gift, the client is likely to feel uncertain and uncomfortable, as well. If you sense that a client may be planning to give you a gift, plan how you will respond, even to the point of rehearsing what you will say.

Sexual Relationships

In terms of sexual relationships with clients, ethical standards are clear: Sex with a current client is unethical. This is specifically prohibited by the ethical standards of psychologists, psychiatrists, social workers, marriage and family therapists, and counselors. Further, sex does not merely mean sexual intercourse. Rather, it is any form of intimate physical contact, such as kissing or fondling (Bouhoutsos et al., 1983; Lamb, Catanzaro, & Moorman, 2004).

When evaluated in terms of the problems with dual relationships listed previously, it is apparent that sex is such a powerful motivating factor that it is impossible to be objective about it. A client's right to make autonomous decisions would certainly be limited by a therapist who made a sexual advance. The therapist's elevated power position, combined with the fact that the client expects the therapist to act in a fiduciary capacity, make it virtually impossible for a client to make an autonomous decision regarding sexual involvement. Pope (1985) found that clients who have engaged in sex with their therapists respond in ways similar to incest victims, feeling a sense of betrayal of trust, role confusion, guilt, and so on.

In addition to the fact that clients have clearly diminished capacities to make autonomous decisions in matters of sexual relationships with therapists, it is also virtually impossible for a therapist to be objective about sex with clients. While clinicians might rationalize that sexual involvements are therapeutic for patients, sexual motives are so powerful that they invariably contaminate clinical judgment. While the process of distinguishing clinical from personal issues is always a concern in therapy, the consequences of being wrong are especially severe when sexual matters are concerned.

An area of greater confusion and disagreement relates to sex with former clients. Whereas it is generally agreed that sexual contact with a current client represents an unethical dual relationship, the issue becomes more complex after termination. One line of reasoning argues that a prohibition against sex with a former client restricts the client's autonomy. That is, to prohibit an individual from having sexual contact with his or her former therapist implies that, by the mere fact of having been a client, that individual has sacrificed his or her right to make autonomous decisions. Proponents of such a view would say that prohibition of sexual contact with a former client does not speak very highly of our attitudes towards our clients' decision-making ability and/or our view of the effectiveness of therapy.

Another line of reasoning is, "Once a client, always a client." Such a position holds that the same factors that make sex with a current client unethical would also apply to a former client. That is, just because a client has ended treatment, there is no evidence that he or she will immediately develop an objective and symmetrical view of the therapist, nor does it seem likely that the therapist would immediately become completely objective in his or her view of the client. In addition, unpublished data cited by the Ethics Committee of the American Psychological Association (1988) suggest that not only do clients create an internalized "image" of their therapist but also that the vividness and use of this image after termination is correlated with measures of improvement. The same source cites research to show that even in successfully terminated therapies, there tends to be a "gradual working through of the unresolved transference issues with passage of time following the treatment" and that the 5- to 10-year period following therapy would seem to be a critical time in the posttherapeutic development.

The various professional associations and state licensing boards have struggled and continue to struggle with the issue of sex with former clients (Sell, Gottlieb, & Schoenfield, 1986). Some ethical codes have been revised to accommodate the current emphasis on this issue. The current psychiatric version of the *Principles of Medical Ethics* (American Psychiatric Association, 2001) has added the following statement: "Sexual activity with a current or former patient is unethical" (§ 2.1).

The *Ethical Principles of Psychologists and Code of Conduct* (American Psychological Association, 2002) states that

(a) Psychologists do not engage in sexual intimacies with former clients/patients for at least two years after cessation or termination of therapy.

(b) Psychologists do not engage in sexual intimacies with former clients/patients even after a two-year interval except in the most unusual circumstances. Psychologists who engage in such activity after the two years following cessation or termination of therapy and of having no sexual contact with the former client/patient bear the burden of demonstrating that there has been no exploitation, in light of all relevant factors, including (1) the amount of time that has passed since therapy terminated; (2) the nature, duration, and intensity of the therapy; (3) the circumstances of termination; (4) the client's/patient's personal history; (5) the client's/patient's current mental status; (6) the likelihood of adverse impact of the client/patient; and (7) any statements or actions made by the therapist during the course of therapy suggesting or inviting the possibility of a posttermination sexual or romantic relationship with the client/patient. (Standard 10.08)

The *Code of Ethics and Standards of Practice* of the American Counseling Association (1995) holds counselors to essentially identical standards (§ A.7).

As noted by Knapp and VandeCreek (2003), Section 10.06 of the American Psychological Association ethics code (2002) has added the provision that it is an ethical violation for a psychologist to initiate a romantic relationship with close relatives or friends of clients or patients.

As noted earlier, the AAMFT *Code of Ethics* (2001) states, "Sexual intimacy with former clients is likely to be harmful and is therefore prohibited for two years following the termination of therapy or last professional contact. In an effort to avoid exploiting the trust and dependency of clients, marriage and family therapists should not engage in sexual intimacy with former clients after the two years following termination or last professional contact. Should therapists engage in sexual intimacy with former clients following two years after termination or last professional contact, the burden shifts to the therapist to demonstrate that there has been no exploitation or injury to the former client or to the client's immediate family" (§ 1.5).

The code of ethics of the National Association of Social Workers (1999) states, "Social workers should not engage in sexual activities or sexual contact with former clients because of the potential for harm to the client. If social workers engage in conduct contrary to this prohibition or claim that an exception to this prohibition is warranted because of extraordinary circumstances, it is social workers—not their clients—who assume the full burden of demonstrating that the former client has not been exploited, coerced, or manipulated, intentionally or unintentionally" (§ 1.09c).

We support an extremely conservative view regarding sex with former clients. While a clinician could make a case that such involvement is ethically and clinically acceptable in a certain case, we believe that, in virtually all cases, there are so many factors that could complicate the judgment of both individuals involved that the chances for exploitation or restriction of autonomy are extremely high. We consider it very wise, therefore, for the clinician to adopt the position of "Once a client, always a client."

GENERAL GUIDELINES

Although it would be difficult to address every potential dual relationship, we offer some general considerations for avoiding problematic dual relationships:

1. Any type of sexual contact with clients is unethical, as is conducting a professional relationship with a close friend, family member, coworker, or other person in a similarly close or intimate role.
2. For ethical (and legal) reasons, the clinician would be wise to adopt the position that sexual intimacies with a former client should always be avoided.
3. The fulfillment of personal needs should be subordinate to the needs of the client. It is understandable that therapists derive emotional satisfaction of various sorts from their interactions with their clients. For the most part, such needs as those to be helpful and effective are appropriate. Therapists' other needs, such as needs for affection, emotional support, control, sexual gratification, or status should not be a part of the therapeutic context. Overtly or covertly using clients to meet such needs is counter-therapeutic.
4. Therapists must ensure that they have options outside of their treatment relationships for meeting their own emotional and physical needs. A therapist whose social outlets are too limited is very likely to rely too heavily on his or her clients for emotional fulfillment. The likelihood of making ill-advised clinical decisions or making inappropriate demands on a client is thus significantly increased.
5. There are a few "early warning" signs that a therapist might be attempting to meet inappropriate needs with a client. These include an inordinate level of self-disclosure, excessive in spite of one's "better judgment"; the eager anticipation of sessions; particular clients' wishes to prolong sessions or the course of treatment despite having accomplished the major goals of therapy; and wishes (or actions) to please, impress, or punish the client.

6. When in doubt, consult trusted associates. Dual relation-
    ship issues are among those about which it is most difficult
    to be objective, so therapists should not hesitate to obtain
    consultation and should be receptive to the feedback re-
    ceived.

Chapter 7

PATERNALISM:
EXERCISING POWER JUDICIOUSLY AND
PROMOTING CLIENT AUTONOMY

Consider the case of a private practitioner who sees an elderly widower for an initial interview. The client states that he has been communicating with Barbra Streisand and that, through the radio, she has told him to give his life savings to charity. Should the therapist take steps to have a conservator appointed, that is, to have this man declared incompetent to manage his own funds? Should the therapist notify the client's family, regardless of his stated preferences? Should the therapist simply discuss the pros and cons of the intended action?

Consider an additional case: An adult client tells the therapist that she has been hoarding her antidepressant medication because she is thinking of killing herself. She mentions that she is only sharing this information because she knows the rules of confidentiality. Should the therapist take steps toward emergency commitment?

The preceding cases illustrate a conflict, commonly experienced in clinical practice, between the principle of autonomy and the principle of beneficence. As we have noted earlier, and as described by many writers in both mental health and philosophy (e.g., Beauchamp & Childress, 2001; Levine & Lyon-Levine, 1984), the principle of autonomy underscores human beings' right to determine their own goals because it treats individual freedom as a crucial component of human affairs. The implication of this in clinical work is that therapist and client enter into a contractual relationship as two equals. The principle of autonomy implies that the client is treated as an independent agent, whose own goals are paramount, and that the therapist should help the client define and achieve those goals. In contrast, the principle of beneficence underscores the promotion of human welfare as an ultimate good. Acting in accord with this principle means that persons can sometimes be forced to do what is in their best interests. The implication of this principle in clinical practice is that practitioners' perceptions of the best interests of the client may take precedence over clients' wishes. This is typically referred to as paternalistic intervention. The reasoning behind this is that the practitioner has the professional knowledge and judgment to know what is best for the client regardless of the client's wishes much as a parent has for a child.

A clinician can take a number of actions which would be considered paternalistic. Hospitalizing a mentally ill or suicidal patient against his or her will, revealing confidential information to a family member to protect a client, and withholding diagnostic or treatment information from a client would all be considered paternalistic acts if carried out because the therapist believed that this was in the client's best interests and that the client would have preferred another course of action. In all these cases, the practitioner has made a decision in what he or she thinks is the client's best interests, in spite of the client's preferences to the contrary.

This chapter deals with various aspects of paternalism. The first section discusses some of the general ethical issues relevant to the beneficence-autonomy dimension. Several clinical situations in which the question of paternalism is especially relevant are then described. Finally, some guidelines are presented to help the clinician structure his or her decision making regarding paternalism.

ETHICAL ISSUES RELATED TO PATERNALISM

The codes of ethics of the various mental health disciplines make general reference to situations in which a clinician can appropriately act paternalistically. Thus, they imply that there may be contexts in which acting paternalistically is justified ethically. On the other hand, a number of explicit statements in the codes of ethics urge the practitioner to be diligent in safeguarding various aspects of autonomy, such as obtaining informed consent and up-holding clients' rights to control release of information. For ex-ample, the *Code of Ethics* of the National Association of Social Workers (1999) states specifically that "Social workers respect and promote the right of clients to self-determination and assist clients in their efforts to identify and clarify their goals. Social workers may limit clients' right to self-determination when, in the social workers' professional judgment, clients' actions or potential actions pose a serious, foreseeable, and imminent risk to themselves or others" (§ 1.02).

These standards are all based on a respect for clients as indi-viduals who can make their own decisions and act in their own best interests. The clear implication of these standards is that the clients' right to autonomy is the overriding principle. While the prac-titioner may be ethical in acting paternalistically, the situations in which he or she does so must be well justified.

The following sections discuss paternalism in clinical settings and situations in which we believe the therapist may appropriately act to restrict the client's autonomy in some way. Such situations include those in which the client must be protected, in which soci-ety must be protected from the client, and in which there may be justification for withholding diagnostic or treatment information from the client.

PROTECTION OF THE CLIENT

Incompetence or Disability

As mentioned previously, the client should be afforded the maximum autonomy possible. However, at times, clients may dis-play some form of disability that indicates that the practitioner's judgment should override the client's. There is little ethical ambi-guity in the more obvious cases of clients who are so severely im-paired because of thought disorder, mood disorder, or organic brain syndrome that they would be in immediate danger of self-harm. In such cases, the clinician should intervene to hospitalize the client, notify family members, or take some other action to pro-tect the client's well-being, regardless of the patient's preferences. However, the question remains: At what level of disability is the practitioner justified in limiting the client's decision-making options? In the preceding vignette concerning the man who believed he was commanded to give his money to charity, does the level of impairment justify notifying a family member, attempting to have the client declared incompetent, or taking some other step to limit the client's freedom?

In making a decision to take a paternalistic step, the practitioner should consider a number of questions. The reader may find it useful to see if the following guidelines provide direction regarding how to deal with the client in the vignette just mentioned.

1. *What is the disabling condition that you feel justifies paternalism?* The practitioner should be able to document the reasons the client cannot make his or her own decision. It is not enough to state that the client has "poor judgment." There should be some identifiable condition, such as schizophrenia or dementia, that limits the client's decision-making ability.

2. *Are there legal guidelines?* The practitioner needs to be aware of prevailing laws and court decisions, particularly statutes regarding the conditions under which involuntary commitment is mandated. Further, the practitioner should know, or be able to find, the statutory definition of competence. Competence to make contracts, competence to stand trial, and competence to administer one's own financial affairs are, for example, common domains in which statutory limitations exist. These limitations vary by state and can be located by reviewing state law and/or consulting a knowledgeable attorney.

3. *What negative effects would occur if you did not take paternalistic action?* If the client is only likely to make an unwise decision, paternalism becomes harder to justify. However, if failure to act were likely to result in death or serious harm, then paternalistic action would become more justifiable.

4. *Is a less controlling option available?* It may be possible to deal with the issue in a way that safeguards the client's autonomy, possibly in a clinically beneficial manner. For instance, if there is concern about whether the client can care for himself or herself, rather than immediately begin-

ning commitment proceedings, it may be desirable to discuss available options with the client and come up with a mutually satisfactory solution. In the case of the elderly client discussed previously, less controlling actions might include the following: The therapist may ask the client for permission to include the family in sessions to discuss the proper handling of his finances, or the therapist could vigorously encourage the client to wait until a thorough discussion had taken place before acting.

Suicide

Good clinical practice suggests that the clinician pay attention to signs that predict suicide and act accordingly; the clinician could be guilty of professional negligence if he or she overlooks such signs (Bongar, 1991; Swenson, 1986). However, consider the case in which a client does not have a disabling mental condition that would inhibit his or her decision-making ability, seems rational and objective, and yet shows evidence of suicidal intent. Does the practitioner have an obligation to try to stop such a client from committing suicide in such a situation?

Philosophically and ethically speaking, a case could be made that under appropriate circumstances the right to commit suicide is part of the individual's right to autonomy. A number of writers (e.g., Szasz, 1986) have made such a point. On the other hand, suicide is an irrevocable step, driven by complex motivation. This makes it difficult to determine whether an individual is actually making a free, autonomous decision to commit suicide.

It is also difficult to conceive of very many clinicians who, even if they philosophically believe that suicide is an individual's right, could allow a client to leave their office intending suicide. Such behavior would likely be inconsistent with most clinicians' personal ethical frameworks. In addition, there is something clinically meaningful about a patient's disclosure of suicidal intentions, and the clinician must balance his or her ethical and legal obligations with a clinical awareness. The clinical significance of a client's telling a therapist (who is obviously committed to preserving life) of his or her desire to end life must be carefully considered. Indeed, as Hoffman (1979) has provocatively argued, it may be clinically inappropriate to respond to a patient's disclosure of suicidal intentions with a paternalistic intervention such as beginning commitment proceedings, in that this may deprive the patient of a therapeutic opportunity to actively choose to live.

These issues are obviously quite complex. In addition to the ethical decision about "allowing" a client to commit suicide (or not taking steps to prevent it), there is a legal aspect to the issue. Ethical codes and legal case precedent make it clear that therapists are not only permitted to act paternalistically in the interests of preserving their clients' lives, but they could be considered professionally negligent if they fail to take any steps at all (Berman & Cohen-Sandler, 1983; Cohen & Mariano, 1982). If, in the clinician's best professional judgment, the issue can be dealt with clinically and nonpaternalistically without undue risk to the patient's life, then he or she is usually justified in proceeding clinically. However, if the clinician believes that the patient represents a serious suicide risk, then some appropriate action must be taken or the clinician will be acting negligently. As Bongar (1991) has usefully pointed out, clinical, legal, and ethical considerations are tightly interwoven in treatment of the suicidal individual.

Finally, we should note that the principles of ethical reasoning applicable to effective clinical work with the suicidal patient apply as well to treatment decisions regarding those who have severe anorexia (Werth et al., 2003) or self-injurious symptoms (e.g., White, McCormick, & Kelly, 2003).

PROTECTION OF OTHERS

At times a practitioner's obligations to clients may be secondary to his or her societal obligations. However, it is not technically paternalism when a practitioner intervenes to keep a client from hurting someone else; defining an intervention as paternalistic implies that the practitioner is acting in the best interests of the client, not protecting others. Still, it requires only a small stretch of the concept to argue that, in fact, the therapist does help the patient by removing some of his or her freedom to act violently toward others. In addition, of course, the therapist acts to protect third parties who may be potential victims. Some have argued that the concept should not be stretched this far—in fact, society should not expect therapists to do detective work in addition to psychological healing (e.g., Bersoff, 1976). Nonetheless, because the demands made on practitioners in such cases are similar to those placed on them when a paternalistic action is being considered, a discussion of protection of others is appropriate here.

Much has been written about clinicians' legal obligations to protect others from the actions of a client (e.g., Cohen & Mariano, 1982; Kaufman, 1991; Knapp & VandeCreek, 1982). Here, we will present a brief summary of relevant legal issues, followed by a discussion of some of the important ethical considerations.

Violence

As noted earlier in Chapter 4, the *Tarasoff* decision (*Tarasoff v. Board of Regents of the University of California,* 1976) established the obligation of the therapist to protect potential victims of their clients' violence. While this decision has been interpreted as developing a "duty to warn," such breaching of confidentiality is only one of the options available to the practitioner as part of the broader "duty to protect." Other alternatives include hospitalizing the client, modifying the environment so that danger is reduced (such as requiring the client to get rid of lethal weapons), or bringing the potential victim into therapy to resolve problem issues (Knapp & VandeCreek, 1982).

In most cases, for the "duty to protect" to apply, the practitioner must know (or should have known based on prevailing standards of practice) that a client presents an immediate danger to an identifiable person. If there is a high likelihood of violence but no identifiable victim, then the practitioner's options are limited primarily to hospitalization. Several "negligent release" cases have been brought on the grounds that persons dangerous in general should be confined and treated to protect the community at large (Cohen & Mariano, 1982). For the most part, however, court decisions have found therapists negligent more for failure to assess their patients' past histories of violent and/or dangerous behavior than for their inability to predict dangerousness or violent behavior in the future (Appelbaum, 1985). On the other hand, courts have also decided that failure to take action in response to what should have been evidence of violent tendencies is negligent or incompetent (e.g., *Peck v. The Counseling Service of Addison County,* 1985; *Petersen v. State,* 1983).

It is difficult to arrive at a single prevailing standard emerging from the various cases that have followed *Tarasoff.* Outcomes are often contradictory or inconsistent. Felthous (1989) has made the point that the states must enact statutes clearly delineating therapists' responsibilities with regard to dangerous clients. At least 16 states have enacted statutes which have limited the therapist's *Tarasoff* obligations in various ways (Kaufman, 1991).

In summarizing state statutes and case law, it is safe to say that clinicians have an obligation to be aware of any potential for violence on the part of their clients, to consider any past incidents of violence, and to take justifiable steps that are in the best interests of both clients and potential victims. If the client is not committable by prevailing statutes, then the best strategy available to the practitioner may be to maintain the therapeutic relationship and attempt to work on the issues in that context.

Physical and Sexual Abuse

All 50 states have statutes mandating reporting of suspected physical or sexual abuse of a minor (Butz, 1985). If the survey of psychologists conducted by Haas, Malouf, and Mayerson (1986) is representative of other mental health professions, practitioners seem well aware of this requirement. Given the number of times that mandatory reporting questions arise, it is important that clinicians know the prevailing statutes in their jurisdictions. It is particularly important that the clinician know (or be able to find) the pertinent definitions of such terms as physical and sexual abuse, incest, and molestation because knowledge of these definitions is critical in helping a practitioner make a decision as to appropriate action in a given situation.

Ethical Considerations in Protecting Others

Although it appears that practitioners commonly know their legal obligations in the circumstances described previously, obeying the law does not necessarily guarantee that the clinician will be acting ethically. A number of ethical concerns should be addressed by the clinician in the process of defining appropriate actions. The first of these relates to breaching confidentiality. Given prevailing legal requirements and precedents, it may seem that the practitioner is more likely to avoid malpractice suits by routinely reporting any potential violence or any suspected physical or sexual abuse, especially because statutes typically grant immunity from liability to anyone who reports suspected abuse in good faith. Unfortunately, this strategy has ethical shortcomings. Specifically, given our tendency to overpredict violence, a reporting policy that is too liberal may violate the rights of confidentiality of many individuals who are likely to harm no one, as well as potentially to waste the resources of child protection agencies. In fact, the reporting process may damage reputations and relationships. Such concerns must be counterbalanced against the clinician's legal and ethical obligations to protect innocent parties.

Consequently, we recommend that practitioners consider the ethical, as well as the legal, ramifications of their decisions and assiduously avoid a "knee-jerk" reporting strategy. Practitioners should report what they are required to report to protect others, and no more. Consultation with other professionals would obviously prove valuable in questionable situations.

Another significant ethical consideration relates to a major theme in this chapter, namely the importance of safeguarding client autonomy. Even when a decision is made to breach confidentiality or override client desires in another way, there may be means of increasing the client's sense of self-direction. For instance, many clinicians give clients the option of reporting physical or sexual abuse themselves, although the clinician must ensure that the report is actually made. Likewise, in cases of potential violence, clients should, when appropriate, participate in the process of deciding how to ensure the safety of the threatened individual. It has even been noted (Beck, 1982) that this involvement may contribute to the patient's remaining in treatment versus dropping out. Only when circumstances permit no other choice should decisions be made without the client's knowledge and participation. For example, if a particular client is so paranoid and out of control that his or her motivation and ability to improve the situation cannot be trusted, the clinician may decide to exclude him or her from the process of protecting others, even if his or her autonomy is restricted in the process.

WITHHOLDING DIAGNOSTIC OR TREATMENT INFORMATION

Possibly the most commonly encountered aspect of paternalism involves withholding information regarding a client's diagnosis or treatment plan. If this information is not made available to clients, their autonomy is reduced. They lack the information required to make such decisions as whether to receive treatment or what form of treatment to participate in. Obviously, this issue overlaps that of informed consent, and much of what is presented in Chapter 5 is relevant here.

Dawson (1981) lists a number of reasons that therapists withhold or distort information. Among these are the client's perceived inability to understand relevant information because of its technical nature, the fact that diagnostic and treatment information is always uncertain in psychotherapy, the client's lack of desire to know, incapacity of the client to be informed, resistance of the therapist, and nonmaleficence (i.e., the therapist's wish to avoid harming the client). In reviewing the justifications for each of these reasons, Dawson concludes that there is typically very little justification for withholding "autonomy-relevant" information or for deceiving clients. Only two situations justify withholding information: when the client's disability prevents him or her from being able to understand or make decisions based on relevant information, or when the practitioner determines that the knowledge would be harmful to the client (e.g., telling a client you think he or she has dementia).

The implication for practice is that clients should be given access to all relevant information unless there is a good reason for it to be withheld. If a client has some incapacity that clearly limits his or her ability to understand or make appropriate decisions, then the clinician has the option, and often the obligation, to withhold information.

With regard to nonmaleficence, it is important that practitioners be very deliberate in defining situations in which full disclosure of information would be countertherapeutic or harmful to the client in some other way. As Dawson mentions, a number of factors can produce positive outcomes in therapy, such as the placebo effect, an optimistic attitude on the part of the therapist, and the therapist's ability to stimulate confidence and trust. To the extent that withholding certain information enhances these factors, doing so may be ethically justifiable. However, at the same time, the clinician should be constantly aware of the client's right to make autonomous decisions and include this factor in his or her decision making, as well.

Further, it is critical that the clinician not confuse nonmaleficence and convenience. That is, the decision to withhold relevant treatment information should be based on avoiding harm to the client rather than on what is easiest for the therapist. Generally, decisions to withhold information tend to result from therapists' concerns that clients will become upset or even leave treatment as a result. Consider, for example, a case in which the therapist believes that treatment will be very lengthy and the client asks, "How long will we need to meet?" A therapist who avoids this question may possibly believe that it would be disturbing to a client to realize that he or she is a "long-term case." Perhaps the therapist believes that there is no effective way to answer the question truthfully. However, the likely motivation in such cases may well be the desire not to commit oneself or get "locked in" to a specific treatment duration. In the former case, paternalistic action is justified on the basis of client welfare. That is, the potentially resistant client may be better able to hear the information at a later time. In the latter case, it is possible that self-interest, rather than paternalism, is the real issue.

Alternatively, consider the case of a therapist who is asked, "Have you ever seen anyone like me before?" and who indeed has not. If the situation is not similar to that discussed in Chapter 3, in which referral or supervision is indicated, then the question of paternalism versus nonmaleficence arises. Telling the client that one is new to his or her problem may undermine faith in treatment (unless it is done in such a way that the client becomes a "team member" and collaborates on treatment). But not revealing such information may be deceptive.

CONCLUSION AND RECOMMENDATIONS

Because paternalism can subtly intrude on clinical practice, practitioners should periodically question themselves (or have colleagues question them) about ways in which the same clinical end could be achieved without sacrificing client autonomy. Perhaps because of a lower frustration tolerance, medicalization of clinical practice, or gradual loss of humility, practitioners can find it easier to "do for" the client instead of facilitating the client's "doing for" himself or herself. We are not advocating abandonment of one's responsibility to clients. Rather, we suggest that periodic attention to this issue is not only of ethical importance, but can lend an elegance and authority to therapy that is not easily achieved any other way.

Chapter 8

LOYALTY CONFLICTS: BALANCING PROFESSIONAL AND ORGANIZATIONAL DEMANDS

Loyalty conflicts may be defined as situations in which a practitioner bears a professional obligation to two or more parties, roles, or functions and these obligations are contradictory in some way. The practitioner is thus in a position of having to establish priorities for professional loyalties and responsibilities. Such conflicts can emerge in both subtle and overt ways. Unfortunately, the ethical standards of the various mental health disciplines offer little specific guidance in terms of practical decision making regarding loyalty conflicts. Beyond fairly general statements such as "Social workers' primary responsibility is to promote the well-being of clients. In general, clients' interests are primary" (NASW, 1999, § 1.01), practitioners are largely left to their own devices.

This chapter is devoted to the question of loyalty conflicts in professional practice. Four general categories of loyalty conflicts are highlighted, along with some of the specific considerations of each. The types of loyalty conflicts to be discussed include conflicts based on difficulty defining the client, conflicts between loyalty to the client and loyalty to one's organization, conflicts between loyalty to the client and appropriate standards of professional practice, and conflicts between loyalty to the client and society (as embodied in law). Last, we consider loyalty conflicts specific to managed care arrangements.

LOYALTY CONFLICTS BASED ON
DIFFICULTY IN DEFINING THE CLIENT

In the simplest case, the client is both the focus of service (e.g., evaluation, therapy) and the source of payment. If these are two different individuals or entities, then the issues become more problematic. Questions arise concerning such issues as ownership of information, rights of confidentiality, and where the practitioner's responsibilities lie when the parties conflict. This problem has been most thoroughly explored with regard to the dilemmas psychologists face when being hired to provide psychological services in the criminal-justice system (see Monahan, 1980).

However, similar problems exist for other professionals and in other aspects of clinical practice. Consider the following example: An attorney contacts a psychotherapist because she has a female client, sole custodian of the children, whose ex-husband is suing for visiting rights. The woman has reason to believe that her ex-husband is emotionally unstable, and her attorney requests that the clinician evaluate the ex-husband and bill the ex-wife. Could information be released about the ex-husband without a signed permission to release information from him? Would he even have access to the results of his own evaluation? Similar questions arise when a business hires a practitioner to provide services to its employees (as with an employee assistance program, or EAP), and even when a parent hires a practitioner to provide services to a minor child. If something revealed by the person receiving services is relevant to the party paying the bill, where do the practitioner's loyalties lie? Another example of such potential conflict is the case of a worker who reveals to her EAP therapist that she is embezzling funds from the company.

In our reading of current ethical standards and available literature, we find little that a practitioner can fall back on to help make decisions in these situations. In the ethical standards of the various mental health professions, the most directly pertinent statement is found in the *Ethical Principles of Psychologists and Code of Conduct* (American Psychological Association, 2002), "When psychologists agree to provide services to a person or entity at the request of a third party, psychologists attempt to clarify at the outset of the service the nature of the relationship with all individuals or organizations involved. This clarification includes the role of the psychologist (e.g., therapist, consultant, diagnostician, or expert witness), an identification of who is the client, the probable uses of the services provided or the information obtained, and the fact that there may be limits to confidentiality" (§ 3.07).

This would suggest that prevention is the best remedy for conflict. That is, practitioners should anticipate the interests and expectations that all parties might have in a particular situation and act in ways that would minimize misunderstanding and failed expectations. What this means specifically varies from situation to situation. In general, the practitioner should assess each party's stake in the action, define the conditions under which the confidentiality of the recipient of services would be breached, and negotiate and obtain agreement on the nature and extent of information sharing. As part of this process, the practitioner may seek consultation regarding the legal aspects of the case. There may be legal constraints within which the practitioner must act and which must be embodied in whatever arrangement is negotiated.

A guiding principle in such negotiations is respect for the privacy of an individual and for the confidentiality of the information that may be shared. This guideline suggests that information should only be revealed to the extent necessary to accomplish the purpose at hand. For example, in a case in which one partner is paying for the evaluation of another, there is no need to share personal information that does not pertain to the question at hand; to share such information would represent an unnecessary violation of an individual's right to privacy (for further elaboration of these issues, see Marsh & Magee, 1997).

To summarize, while ethical guidelines contain little or no specific information about how to resolve dilemmas created by cases involving multiple clients with different demands, we suggest that the practitioner be open about the issues involved, try to anticipate the needs and demands of each party, and negotiate acceptable arrangements in advance. The ideal result of such negotiations would be a plan that reflects the needs of each party, conforms to relevant legal guidelines, and, to the extent possible, protects privacy and confidentiality. A less-than-ideal outcome of such negotiations may bring the practitioner to the conclusion that the parties' different needs cannot be reconciled. In such cases it is better to withdraw as a possible service provider (or to include additional providers) than to accept an impossible contract in the hopes that positions will change (Marsh & Magee, 1997).

LOYALTY TO THE CLIENT VERSUS
LOYALTY TO ONE'S ORGANIZATION

Situations may arise in which the ostensible needs of the client conflict with the needs of the practitioner's employing agency or organization. A number of such situations may occur, such as being requested by an agency director to refer a client to a therapist one does not trust, or being asked to terminate a client who has not paid a bill.

When faced with such questions, what are practitioners' options? Are they ethically bound to honor the client's needs, even if they conflict with the needs of the organization, or can clinicians be ethical and still support such organizational needs, even to the detriment of a client? Again, ethical guidelines make few specific statements relevant to this question. The *Ethical Principles of Psychologists and Code of Conduct* (American Psychological Association, 2002) makes this statement:

> If the demands of an organization with which psychologists are affiliated or for whom they are working conflict with this Ethics Code, psychologists clarify the nature of the conflict, make known their commitment to the Ethics Code, and to the extent feasible, resolve the conflict in a way that permits adherence to the Ethics Code. (Standard 1.03)

While this statement is vague, it clearly does not state the expectation that psychologists obey the ethical principles above all else. In other words, psychologists do not have the obligation to commit professional suicide to uphold the code of ethics. The principle does mandate, however, that psychologists make sure that the issues are clear to concerned individuals, including the fact that there is an ethical concern and that they attempt to comply with the ethical principles as closely as feasible (leaving it up to the psychologist to define "feasible"). The *Code of Ethics and Standards of Practice* of the American Counseling Association (1995) expresses a very similar concept and also adds that counselors should work toward change in the organization "to allow full adherence to the Code of Ethics" (§ H.2.c).

The *Code of Ethics* of the American Association for Marriage and Family Therapy (2001) makes the statement, "If the mandates of an organization with which a marriage and family therapist is affiliated, through employment, contract or otherwise, conflict with the AAMFT Code of Ethics, marriage and family therapists make known to the organization their commitment to the AAMFT Code of Ethics and attempt to resolve the conflict in a way that allows the fullest adherence to the Code of Ethics" (§ 6.1).

The most recent *Code of Ethics* of the National Association of Social Workers (NASW, 1999), makes a stronger statement about this. It says that "Social workers should not allow an employing organization's policies, procedures, regulations, or administrative orders to interfere with their ethical practice of social work. Social workers should take reasonable steps to ensure that their employing organizations' practices are consistent with the *NASW Code of Ethics*" (§3.09d). The word "reasonable" seems to temper the meaning of this section and gives the social worker some flexibility.

Regardless of whether there is a statement in the practitioner's code of ethics, it appears that the practitioner is given some leeway in dealing with situations where there is a conflict between loyalty to one's client and loyalty to one's organization. Following are descriptions of two types of situations in which the practitioner is confronted with such conflicting loyalties.

Loyalty Conflicts Relating to Client Confidentiality

Consider the situation in which a client tells her therapist at a mental health center that she has not been taking the medication prescribed by the staff psychiatrist. Or consider a situation in which a patient at an agency that sets fees on a sliding scale tells the therapist that he makes more money than he initially reported. If proper procedures for providing information necessary to obtain informed consent have been followed (see Chapter 5), then the client has been led to believe that the therapist will maintain complete confidentiality (with the exception of such legal requirements as mandatory reporting). This places the clinician in an ethical conflict regarding whether to reveal confidential information to other members of the organization without the expressed consent of the client. While customary practice allows for some necessary sharing of information when appropriate, clients may, not unreasonably, expect to have their confidences respected.

In dealing with situations such as the ones discussed previously, the clinician does have certain options. The first, of course, would be to anticipate such problems and include specific statements related to them in a consent form signed by the client. Second, the situation can be handled as a clinical issue (e.g., dealing with it as a possible request for limit-setting). Third, the clinician may strongly assert that he or she needs to share the confidential information with the appropriate individual(s) within the organization and try to elicit the patient's consent to do so. If such consent is not forthcoming, the practitioner may decide that effective therapy with the client is impossible under the circumstances (e.g., the client's unwillingness to allow coordination among clinical personnel, or personal feelings aroused by the client's deceptiveness). In such a case, termination or transfer may be justifiable.

Conflicts Based On Disagreements With One's Organization

The example cited in the previous section puts loyalty conflicts in a context in which the practitioner supports the organization's policies. What are a clinician's alternatives if he or she feels that the organization, or a representative thereof, is wrong? For instance, the clinician might determine that a client needs long-term therapy while the agency allows only six sessions; or the client clearly needs psychotropic medications and the agency director has a firm antimedication stance. In polling psychologists about a specific instance of this dilemma, Haas et al. (1986) found that the vast majority of psychologists stated that they would refuse to support the organizational policy if they disagreed with it.

It would obviously be ethically unsound for a clinician to support a policy that he or she believed was harmful to the client. Such an action would be contrary to the practitioner's obligation to promote the client's welfare. At the same time, openly disagreeing with the policy may be destructive to the unity of the organization, as well as possibly countertherapeutic for the client. Resolving such a dilemma would require that the clinician exercise a significant amount of diplomacy, working to change the organization's position while not being openly critical of it with the client. The clinician would be wise to spend time trying to understand and clarify both his or her own and the agency's positions, searching for areas of possible compromise. If no mutually satisfactory resolution can be found, then the clinician is forced to make a decision to either support or contradict the organization's position and to deal with the consequences of the decision. This would likely be a no-win situation, so expending considerable effort to arrive at a mutually acceptable resolution of the problem would clearly be worth the time. For example, in the preceding illustration, the clinician might see the client pro bono (at no cost) while advocating for an exception with the director. The alternative of simply discharging the client and immediately picking him or her up again for another six sessions probably would be considered deceptive or manipulative and not contribute to a reasonable resolution. In the second example, the clinician could obviously refer the case to a more appropriate agency, but this leaves the policy unchanged. Perhaps the therapist could initiate a discussion among the staff regarding the wisdom of such an antimedication policy. This might enhance the chances of the director changing his or her mind. This type of dilemma is likely to present itself in the managed care arena, as the dictates of the patient's insurance plan often restrict treatment options although they do not restrict the therapist's obligation to provide treatment. Geraty, Hendren, and Flaa (1992) describe the increasing influence of managed care on the practice of child and adolescent psychiatry, for example, detailing the clinician liability in a managed health care context (*Wickline v. State of California*, 1986), in which ultimate responsibility for the proper treatment of a patient was placed on the treating physician. The insurance company was absolved in a suit of negligence brought by the patient (cf. also, Appelbaum, 1993; also, discussion in Chapter 11).

CONFLICTS BETWEEN LOYALTY TO THE CLIENT AND APPROPRIATE STANDARDS OF PROFESSIONAL PRACTICE

At times clinicians may feel caught between what they believe to be in the best interest of a client and appropriate standards of professional practice. For example, a clinician may be working with a recently divorced woman who is emotionally healthy but who has no vocational skills nor any money to educate herself. For her to qualify for publicly sponsored rehabilitation services, it is necessary to document an emotional disorder of some sort, and the client may ask the therapist to do so. What are the clinician's options and responsibilities in such situations? Is it helpful to diagnose her and thereby help her obtain the money, or is this an abdication of professional responsibility?

To further illustrate, a divorcing client may ask the clinician to come to court and testify that the client is the more effective parent and should be granted custody. Assuming that he or she has not met the spouse and thus can make no comparison, what options are available to the clinician? To accede to the client's wish would violate an important standard of professional practice, in that a practitioner cannot responsibly make comparative statements when he or she has only met one of the spouses.

These conflicts often arise because of conflicting demands for objectivity and advocacy. While standards of professional practice promote objectivity—asserting that clinicians are expected to diagnose accurately, base their clinical recommendations on valid data, and so on—clinicians are frequently seen by their clients as being advocates. Clinicians themselves are often drawn to the client-advocate role. Implied in this role can be pressures on the clinician to compromise professional standards in the service of client needs.

Although there is certainly room for debate regarding whether to compromise standards of professional practice, our contention is that these standards should be compromised very rarely, if ever. There are several reasons for a stringently conservative view regarding this. The first is purely ethical. For example, in the rehabilitation eligibility case cited above, a lie is being requested. Lying is inherently unethical, even though arguments for "tempering the truth" can and have been made. The burden of proof is obviously on a practitioner who distorts the truth to show why such an action is justified.

The second reason a conservative view is preferred involves the credibility of the mental health professions. If individuals freely compromise their professional judgment, even for what seem to be good reasons, the overall effect is a reduction in the public's trust of mental health specialists as objective professionals. Increased stringency in insurance company reimbursements and decreased influence of mental health professionals in court, among other outcomes, may result.

Clinical considerations comprise the third justification for a conservative stance. While in the short run it may seem appropriate to sacrifice one's standards on behalf of a client, the precedent may have an overall deleterious effect on the therapeutic relationship. The impact of knowing that one's therapist compromised his or her own standards, no matter what the reason, may ultimately prove countertherapeutic. For example, such actions may create the expectation that the clinician will solve all of the client's problems, thus removing the responsibility for problem solving from the client.

With the above in mind, what should a clinician do if confronted with a conflict between ethical standards and client needs? First, clinicians should honestly assess their motivations. Is this truly an ethical conflict, or is there some other motivation, such as desiring to avoid alienating a client or funding source, securing reimbursement, taking the path of least resistance, wanting to be admired, or the like? Second, the clinician should explore alternatives. Are there other, more professionally honest, ways of dealing with the problem? Third, the clinician should consider the negative impacts of compromising standards—on the client, on the relationship, and on psychotherapeutic practice in general. Only if the motivation is truly ethical, there are no alternatives, and the benefits heavily outweigh the costs should the clinician consider sacrificing professional standards.

For example, the clinician in this case could help the client search for a different rehabilitation program. It should also be noted that telling the truth in this type of case preserves one's credibility with the agency. Alternatively, one could, without distorting the truth, advocate for the patient with the agency, and/or describe the likely results of failure to obtain the rehabilitation service. In the custody-evaluation case, the most professionally honest course would be to report only what one knows and to suggest appropriate, unbiased evaluations.

CONFLICTS BETWEEN LOYALTY TO THE CLIENT AND THE LAW

The practitioner may feel himself or herself in a bind when confronted by a conflict between the obligation to obey the law and duty to the client. Such binds may be created by cases of mandatory reporting, duty to warn, responding to subpoenas, and related issues (see Chapters 4 and 7). If the clinician believes that obeying the law may not be in the client's best interest, then a true dilemma is created.

In deciding how to resolve such dilemmas, the practitioner could choose the safest course, always obeying the law. As long as the law is clear, well understood, and appropriately followed, such a course may be justifiable. However, it is incumbent on the practitioner not to play it so safe that confidentiality is unnecessarily breached. This might occur, for example, through reporting clinical information or responding to subpoenas when such action is not justified. For instance, it may assuage the practitioner's anxiety to report to the authorities or family members any hint of suicide or physical aggressiveness raised in therapy. However, this is inappropriate unless the practitioner believes that the behavior is highly likely to occur. Various sources (e.g., Committee on Professional Practice and Standards, 2003; DeKraii & Sales, 1984; Knapp & VandeCreek, 1982) describe the conditions under which confidentiality may be breached.

Other practitioners may believe that slavish obedience to the law is not ethical (that good client care may be compromised by "overconforming"). The clinician, for instance, may believe it inappropriate to report a case of sexual molestation, thinking that doing so would alienate the client and interrupt the therapeutic process. Such noncompliance is very risky for a number of reasons. First, when the law establishes the conditions for violating a client's right to confidentiality, it is usually done to protect the security of innocent individuals. If the clinician does not abide by legal requirements, he or she is, in effect, assuming responsibility for the well-being of potential victims; if something does happen and someone is hurt, the clinician bears the moral (and legal) responsibility. Given the inaccuracy of predicting behavior and the tendency to believe a client's assertions that any inappropriate behavior will not be repeated, the risk of disobeying the law is significant.

Another risk in disobeying the law is that of making a clinical mistake. The credibility and professionalism of a clinician who violates a legal requirement is likely to be compromised, and, unfortunately, many clients would capitalize on this compromised position in service of their own needs. Also, by agreeing to keep a secret, the clinician may effectively buffer the client from dealing with the consequences of his or her own behavior and thus allow avoidance of responsibility.

In deciding whether to obey legal requirements, the clinician would thus be wise to adopt a very stringent standard and to consider a number of aspects, only some of which are the same as in the preceding section. First, the practitioner should assess his or her own motivations. Is the temptation to disregard the law truly based on the best interest of the client, or are there other motivations, such as a desire not to make the client angry or a desire to avoid legal procedures? Second, is it clear that disobedience to the law is obviously the best course clinically? Third, is the clinician willing to accept any consequences that result if the legal disobedience is brought to light? Although taking such action may be quite difficult, such a decision-making process may reduce the number of conflicts between the professional's personal standards and the perceived demands of the law.

LOYALTY CONFLICTS IN MANAGED CARE

As noted in Chapter 4, managed mental health care contracts insert a third party into the clinical relationship. These systems regulate the use of health care with "gatekeepers" and review the care provided to individual patients. They reserve the right to deny payment for care they deem medically unnecessary or excessive (Appelbaum, 1993). It is likely that the trend toward such arrangements will increase.

In addition to the financial, legal, and clinical concerns which managed care raises, there are a number of ethical concerns with which the clinician must deal. These concerns have been discussed in the literature (e.g., Lowman, 1991). This section will highlight some of the major ethical issues and will attempt to provide some recommendations for practitioners struggling with these problems.

A primary ethical concern in dealing with the managed mental health care system is whether clients are able to receive mental health care that is appropriate to their needs and of sufficient intensity and duration. The ethical conflict centering on the financial incentive for reducing care is difficult to resolve. What responsibilities does the clinician incur when an external body approves and directs a client's treatment and when that external body may have incentives for limiting the amount of treatment provided? First, the clinician has the responsibility to ensure that he or she has sought approval for an appropriate level of care and has provided the necessary documentation. In other words, the therapist must play by the rules if he or she has already agreed to do so.

Second, if the managed care organization refuses to approve treatment that the clinician believes is necessary, the clinician should pursue the case through all necessary appeal steps. This is not only an ethically appropriate stance, but it may be legally prudent as well. The *Wickline* case (*Wickline v. State of California*, 1986) is illustrative in this regard. The clinician (in this case not a therapist) was held liable for failing to protest the HMO's denial of treatment to a man who later died from the illness. Third, the clinician has the ethical and often legal obligation to continue services even though payment may be terminated. The therapeutic obligation supersedes the financial contract.

The pressure to join particular managed mental health care plans is one that practitioners will increasingly face. Haas and Cummings (1991) discuss the issues prospective providers should consider. They urge that prospective providers know exactly what the plan involves and what constraints will be imposed. Specific questions concern the following:

1. *Who takes the risks?* If the practitioner takes the financial risk for services exceeding what was predicted (as is the case in HMO arrangements), there may be a temptation to limit services inappropriately.
2. *How much does the plan intrude into the patient/provider relationship?* As opposed to traditional fee-for-service arrangements, managed care systems involve more intrusion into the therapeutic relationship. At the minimum this typically involves a much greater intrusion into confidentiality than in traditional arrangements (e.g., through preauthorization requirements, chart reviews). Practitioners must be able to balance loyalty to their patients with responsibilities as "agents" of the mental health care carrier.
3. *What provisions exist for appealing adverse rulings?* The clinician should consider the plan's options for extending

treatment beyond the typical length of service approved by the plan.

4. *Are there referral resources if patient needs exceed plan benefits?* Although there is an obligation in all the mental health professions to avoid abandonment, there are practical limitations in terms of how many low-fee or no-fee cases a practitioner can afford to carry. The ethical clinician must consider how to avoid abandoning patients without going bankrupt (Appelbaum, 1993).

5. *Is the plan open to provider input?* If there is no mechanism for the practitioner to provide feedback to the plan managers, then it is hard to characterize his or her role as that of a professional independently or autonomously treating patients. The clinician can have no assurance that the plan managers are indeed interested in delivering quality care, although this can be hoped for.

6. *Does the plan clearly inform policyholders about the limits of their benefits?* This is an issue of informed consent, but it is one which the therapist would be well advised to raise with prospective clients before they enter a treatment relationship.

Managed care arrangements are not inherently unethical and may, in fact, reduce certain ethical concerns (e.g., the temptation to provide excessive services because one is reimbursed for them). Nonetheless, managed care systems do raise ethical problems, and the clinician involved with such systems would be wise to anticipate and deal with them in advance.

Chapter 9

ETHICAL RELATIONSHIPS WITH COLLEAGUES

No mental health professional practices in isolation. Whether it is consultation with colleagues to improve the treatment of a particularly complex case, discussing professional norms, or simply becoming aware of how colleagues handle particular issues, we all spend a considerable portion of our professional lives in dialogue with colleagues in our own and related mental health professions. Additionally, our practices intertwine: We get backup or emergency coverage from our colleagues, and provide same; we make referrals to colleagues, and they choose us for referrals. In all these activities the mental health professions are largely self-regulating. That is, a substantial portion of the responsibility for maintaining professional standards falls on professionals themselves. This means that mental health practitioners have an ethical obligation not only to monitor their own behavior and take steps to deal with conflicts or personal problems that interfere with professional effectiveness, but also to deal with colleagues who appear to be practicing at a substandard level. When we ourselves are not functioning effectively or are making ethical errors, colleagues are likewise obligated to take action. The codes of all the mental health professionals underscore practitioners' obligation to confront, when appropriate, their colleagues' questionable behavior. Indeed, ethical (or unethical) behavior does not just affect our patients or clients, but it also affects our colleagues and the public's trust in our professions.

If professionals do not effectively manage to self-regulate, outside bodies such as government agencies or the courts will be more likely to do so for us. On the other hand, development of a vigilante culture in which professionals suspiciously monitor each other is a distasteful prospect. A reasonable balance is needed. These notions thus imply that, whether one is on the receiving or the giving end of professional peer scrutiny, one has the obligation to treat colleagues (members of one's own and related disciplines) responsibly.

Consider the following examples:

Example 1. Reading about the progress of a trial in which a colleague is providing expert testimony, a forensic practitioner believes that his colleague is distorting and misrepresenting relevant facts about the cases in which he is involved.

Example 2. A female client of a therapist tells him about her previous male therapist who would hug her at the end of each session, and during the hug would press against her for a very lengthy period of time. The client is distressed about this.

These examples illustrate situations in which a mental health professional is concerned about a colleague's behavior: The questionable behavior may be a result of incompetence, impairment, lack of ethical awareness, or deliberate violation of professional standards. The code of ethics of various mental health disciplines do touch on such situations, but in ways that offer little specific guidance. Should those affected by the professional's behavior be alerted, or should a regulatory body be informed? Should the professional in question be confronted, or should the problem be discussed with other colleagues first? Not only is there confusion and stress among mental health practitioners about the most appropriate response to suspected unethical or substandard practices, but there is also concern about the consequences of failure to respond.

In a sense, the present chapter focuses on a sort of etiquette of collegial relationships. Many of the issues to be raised are matters of prudence and tact necessary in the upholding of sound ethical standards. Although the obligation to confront colleagues is present or implied in a number of ethics codes, the *processes* of so doing are not always entirely clear. In addition, it is frequently not clear what the cost/benefit ratio of such confrontation or consultation might be. The cultural norms against "tattling" or "whistleblowing" are quite strong, and, paradoxically, allegations of a "culture of silence" among professionals is one source of pressure for ever-tighter controls over the health care professions. In light of these issues, professional competence in self-regulation increases in importance. Fundamentally, we feel that the mental health professions' ethical culture is much more a result of collegial and individual professional decisions than legislative, judicial, or consumer pressure.

Is the Colleague's Behavior Unethical or Impaired?

Unethical behavior can be the result of a number of factors. At times it may be motivated by conscious and manipulative motives (e.g., money, power). Unethical behavior can also be the result of ignorance. In many cases unethical professional behavior is driven by factors we would consider to be psychological impairment, such as alcoholism, depression, or marital conflict. Regardless of motivation or level of consciousness, however, one must deal in some way with the unethical behavior of colleagues.

Dealing with the problem begins with the elimination of denial. Abuse of alcohol and other drugs, psychological disorders, burnout, and other impairments affect mental health professionals just as they do the general public (VandenBos & Duthie, 1986). Often the impaired or distressed* professional's colleagues will be in the best position to confront the difficulties. It is useful to remember that impaired professionals are frequently skillful at denying and rationalizing their difficulties. The evidence available on this topic (e.g., Freudenberger, 1982; Norcross & Prochaska, 1983;

---

*Many experts distinguish between *impaired* professionals, who have disorders which harm their work, and *distressed* professionals, who are emotionally upset but who maintain an adequate level of work (VandenBos & Duthie, 1986).

VandenBos & Duthie, 1986) suggests that mental health professionals have difficulty admitting that they need help and often believe that they are simply situationally troubled.

The mental health professions' codes of ethics promote different levels of activity with regard to intervention. At the most "activist" level, the psychiatrists' code of ethics indicates that "It is ethical, even encouraged, for another psychiatrist to intercede" when a psychiatrist who because of mental illness jeopardizes the welfare of patients (American Psychiatric Association, 2001, § 2.4). According to the American Psychological Association (2002):

(a) Psychologists refrain from initiating an activity when they know or should know that there is a substantial likelihood that their personal problems will prevent them from performing their work-related activities in a competent manner.

(b) When psychologists become aware of personal problems that may interfere with their performing work-related duties adequately, they take appropriate measures, such as obtaining professional consultation or assistance, and determine whether they should limit, suspend, or terminate their work-related duties. (Standard 2.06)

Counselors are also "alert to the signs of impairment, seek assistance for problems, and, if necessary, limit, suspend, or terminate their professional responsibilities" (ACA, 1995, § C.2.g).

It is often difficult for distressed professionals to find help, however. Especially if they have reached the senior ranks of the mental health professions, putting themselves in the patient role, much less finding a therapist who can be trusted and respected, may be difficult. Thus, a frequent rationale for avoiding confronting a colleague about questionable behavior—"I'm sure he realizes that he has a problem and is doing something about it"—is unlikely to be true. Further, the comforting notion that professionals' disorders are time limited is without empirical support. Our approach to patients—that treatment can help to restore effective personal and professional functioning—is one we should apply to ourselves.

METHODS OF DEALING WITH IMPAIRED
OR UNETHICAL BEHAVIOR

Beyond hoping that the individual will get himself or herself into treatment, probably the modal response to suspected collegial inappropriate behavior is to do nothing. Another frequent response is to discuss the problem with *other* colleagues without directly contacting the individual about whom there are questions. Third, the behavior may be reported to a formal regulatory body. In many situations, the preferred option is to contact the colleague directly with one's questions or concerns. While this can be a desirable option, it is also extremely difficult (and perhaps even risky) to implement. For example, the colleague may react defensively or even threaten a counteraccusation (and this raises fears in all practitioners because no one feels completely certain of the purity of his or her practice). Not surprisingly, we comfort ourselves with the thought that someone else will eventually do the job, or we hope that we have been misinformed. Even when we do attempt to confront our colleagues, we are poor at giving each other direct feedback (Gary Schoener, personal communication, 1989; Ende, 1983).

GUIDANCE FROM ETHICS CODES
ABOUT COLLEGIAL MISCONDUCT

As noted previously, the various mental health professions' codes endorse differing levels of activism with regard to suspected collegial misconduct. The social workers' code of ethics (NASW, 1999) states, "Social workers should take adequate measures to discourage, prevent, expose, and correct the unethical conduct of colleagues" (§ 2.11a). Similarly, psychiatrists should "strive to expose those physicians deficient in character or competence, or who engage in fraud or deception" (American Psychiatric Association, 2001, § 2). The psychologists' code of conduct endorses direct discussion when appropriate: "When psychologists believe that there may have been an ethical violation by another psychologist, they attempt to resolve the issue by bringing it to the attention of that individual, if an informal resolution appears appropriate and the intervention does not violate any confidentiality rights that may be involved" (American Psychological Association, 2002, § 1.04). According to the American Counseling Association,

"When counselors possess reasonable cause that raises doubts as to whether a counselor is acting in an ethical manner, they take appropriate action" (ACA, 1995, H.2.a). The marriage and family therapists' code of ethics takes a more legalistic approach: "Marriage and family therapists comply with applicable laws regarding the reporting of alleged unethical conduct" (American Association for Marriage and Family Therapy, 2001, § 1.6).

PRACTICAL GUIDANCE ON CONFRONTATION

Regardless of their differing emphases, no professional ethics code prohibits direct confrontation of the colleague about whom one has questions. For guidance in capably and tactfully undertaking such an endeavor, a useful beginning is outlined in a paper by VandenBos and Duthie (1986). These authors make several useful suggestions: Among them, they advise that it is helpful to approach colleagues in a questioning manner, first ascertaining that one has accurate information. It is important not to presume guilt or innocence in these matters. On the other hand, it is important to be frank about one's concerns and, if one believes that a problem exists, to be forthright in recommending that the potentially impaired colleague seek help in remedying the difficulties. The field could benefit from case reports of successful use of this approach and inclusion of this issue in graduate and postgraduate training curricula.

It is commonly assumed that a confrontation involves the face-to-face criticism of a colleague for unethical behavior, but this is not necessarily always the case. A "confrontation" may be as gentle and nonthreatening as raising a tactful question about a colleague's behavior or area of responsibility. It may also take a more indirect form, such as reflecting with a colleague (e.g., "You know, I once had a problem like this, and what I did was. . . ."). Of course, the more indirect the approach, the more one must ensure that the message was indeed received and not denied. Despite the gentleness of the approach, it remains the case that pointing out possible misconduct on the part of a colleague puts one in a precarious position; one risks alienating the colleague regardless of whether (perhaps especially if) one is correct about the misconduct. This implies that the practitioner should weigh the potential costs of confrontation against the possible benefits. Potential costs

include harm to the collegial relationship and the chance of aggra-
vating the situation in some way, such as if the practitioner retali-
ates against a client. The major benefit of confrontation is the
elimination of harmful or unethical practices. One should also
consider the harm that is done to the reputation of the profession if
confrontation is avoided and the harmful practices continue. If
slight but damaging ethical misdeeds are left unchallenged, tolerance of collegial misconduct rapidly leads to perceptions among
laypersons that a profession is cynically self-serving. On the other
hand, constant chiding from one's colleagues can lead to a sort of
competition among professionals to point out each other's wrong-
doing. This state of affairs can escalate into avoidable charges being filed with the state association's or the national association's
ethics committees regarding colleagues' behavior (David Mills, personal communication, 1984).

It is also important to note that the presumption of innocence may be as important as tactfulness in confronting colleagues. Many professional ethical violations may result from
ignorance rather than "willful disregard" of ethical standards
(Keith-Spiegel, 1977). In addition, often the confronting professional has only indirect evidence of the substandard conduct.

Unfortunately, it is common for colleagues questioned about
the ethical appropriateness of their behavior to react defensively.
If the suspected misdeed is serious enough, this defensive reaction
may lead the confronting professional to avoid further direct contact with the individual and instead report concerns to the appropriate regulatory body (i.e., licensing board or ethics committee).
Such an action will not endear one to a colleague whose actions
are questioned, and it is certainly advisable to consider alternatives,
such as offering a chance to "cool off" and pursue the discussion at
a later time, or a suggestion to consult with a respected colleague
for a "second opinion." If these efforts fail, a report to the ethics
committee or licensing board is essential.

One issue to keep in mind is patient confidentiality. This is
particularly a problem when a current client reveals improper behavior by a previous therapist. If the current client requests confidentiality, the prior therapist cannot respond to an inquiry without
breaching confidentiality (although the client can be identified to
the questioned therapist with client's permission). These sorts of
cases are probably best handled by encouraging the client to file a

complaint directly with the appropriate ethics committee or licensing board. However, this raises problems, too, because the client will then have to confront his or her previous therapist. If the client chooses not to do this and refuses to allow his or her identity to be revealed to the prior therapist, despite feelings of frustration and anger, there is nothing further that the ethical therapist can do.

Practitioners in more vulnerable positions, such as trainees or students who are having difficulty with the actions of their superiors, are a special case. Such individuals may fear they could harm their chances for completing training if they come forward with questions about their supervisors' behavior. For psychologists, there is a "statute of limitations" that is somewhat of a protection. That is, the psychologist who is in a training position who wishes to file an ethics charge has a period of 3 years from the date at which the training status is terminated in which the charge can be filed. Psychiatric trainees appear to be somewhat better protected, in that psychiatrists do not impose any "statute of limitations" on ethics charges.

A final consideration concerning confrontation is that of separating one's emotional reactions from one's professional reactions. It is easy to rationalize the misconduct of one's friends and easy to judge too harshly the conduct of one's enemies. Again, weighing the consequences of confrontation against the consequences of the misdeed's continuing is essential in arriving at a balanced conclusion. Evaluating the alternatives to direct confrontation when one is considering the actions of a disliked colleague and considering the usefulness of a gentle inquiry when reviewing the actions of a liked colleague are both appropriate steps.

It is important that the responsible practitioner be aware of resources for the distressed professional. For example, physicians in many states, as well as the American Medical Association nationally, have developed model programs and model statutes for "disabled doctors" (Laliotis & Grayson, 1985).

Many state professional associations now operate "colleague assistance" programs for drug- or alcohol-abusing professionals in recovery.

BEING CONFRONTED BY A COLLEAGUE

Even the best intentioned professional may, for good or poor reasons, find himself or herself confronted by a colleague because of concerns about professional behavior. From an ethical perspective, it is apparent that the practitioner being confronted should consider objectively the nature of the concern being expressed. It is probably obvious to any competent, mature practitioner that it is best to view challenges as opportunities to learn rather than occasions to counterattack. Nonetheless, a few obvious issues in this domain are probably worth emphasizing. Given the natural human tendency to be angry and defensive in such situations, it is likely that one's first response will be to disqualify the message or the messenger in some way, for instance, "How dare he tell me that I have done anything wrong. He's the most arrogant therapist I've ever seen," or "She doesn't know good therapy when she sees it." The person being confronted may be tempted to question the motives of the confronting practitioner, and conceivably the motives may not be honorable or may reflect some personal agenda, such as professional jealousy or personal rivalry. However, the accuser's motives are technically irrelevant, and the confronted practitioner should attempt to set motives aside and deal with the content of the concern. The relevant question is whether there is any substance to the issue raised. The psychologists' code offers the chance to file a countercomplaint of frivolous charges (undoubtedly the other professional ethics bodies would entertain similar charges if merited), but this can only be done after the initial issue has been resolved, so it is best to do this with grace and not inflame one's accuser no matter how much he or she seems to deserve it.

Once the practitioner has succeeded in separating the message from the messenger, the next step is to assess the legitimacy of the concern. Was the action unethical, illegal, unwise, or inappropriate in some other way? In what ways, if any, did it violate the relevant ethical standards? In what ways, if any, did it violate the law? Was a client or other party harmed in any way? Did the reputation of the profession suffer? In answering such questions, as with many discussed in this book, it may be useful to consult a trusted colleague or even to seek advice from the appropriate ethics, professional standards, or licensing committee. It may also be useful to consider the issue in question in terms of some of the dimensions discussed previously in this book. Specifically, could the practitioner defend what he or she did to a group of peers? In a similar situation, would the practitioner do the same thing again and recommend that others do the same?

If the result of these deliberations is that the practitioner feels that no violation was committed, then he or she may wish to report back to the individual who expressed the concern, stating the process that was employed and the reasons for the decision that was made. If, on the other hand, the practitioner decides that the action in question was in fact inappropriate, then corrective steps should be determined. If a client was harmed, steps must be taken to rectify the harm. There should also be steps taken to ensure that the behavior will never recur. Again, it may be desirable to notify the confronting practitioner of what conclusions were drawn and what remedial steps were taken. Certainly one should document the actions one took in case further accusations emerge.

If the questioned actions are indeed fairly serious, it may be better to submit the problem to the local or national ethics committee for resolution. This is recommended because (a) ethics committees do have as part of their charge an educative function so that they may help a practitioner learn what caused the problem (note the difference between ethics committees and licensing boards, which have the charge to protect the public—they ordinarily are not good sources for advisory opinions); and (b) having the matter resolved formally will prevent an informal resolution being followed by formal charges. It is certainly not unknown for well-meaning therapists to attempt an "informal" resolution that involves recontacting an upset and volatile ex-client who then becomes even more upset by the contact and files formal charges subsequently.

ETHICS COMMITTEES AND LICENSING BOARDS

No practitioner wants to be asked to respond to an ethics committee to explain his or her activities, but many practitioners find themselves in such a situation. Regardless of whether the practitioner considers such a request appropriate, it is wise to deal in advance with issues of defensiveness, hostility, and the like. Whenever possible, it is helpful to think of ethics committees as composed of one's colleagues, rather than being composed of inquisitors. It is helpful to view the process as potentially improving the quality of one's professional work rather than to think of it as a trial in which one side is right and the other wrong. These are idealistic notions, of course; because ethics committee members are human, they sometimes can become overly punitive. And because practitioners questioned about ethics matters are also human, they may become overly defensive and hostile. Nonetheless, a focus on the ultimate point of the enterprise—the well-being of clients—may help to reduce the defensiveness on both sides. Defensiveness by the "complainee" can be particularly damaging to even an innocent professional; it may make the committee suspicious.

Many state ethics committees subscribe to the rules and procedures of the national ethics committee of their parent organization (e.g., many state psychological association ethics committees use the published rules and procedures of the American Psychological Association Ethics Committee; Mills, 1986). It is important to note that for professional association ethics committees, due process is *a* feature but not *the* sole feature in the design of their activities. For example, it is a key feature of due process that a "defendant" be permitted to confront the accuser. For reasons of protecting the (presumably) weaker, complaining client, this is rarely a feature of ethics committees' procedure in hearing charges. Psychologists, for example, frequently conduct the investigation entirely on paper; psychiatrists often have both parties present. Conversely, it is sometimes not obvious to observers why ethics committees keep so much of their activities confidential: Shouldn't the profession at large, or consumers for that matter, know who has been charged with what? Despite these pressures, ethics committees exist to change professionals' appropriate practices and not necessarily to punish the "guilty."

AWARENESS OF OTHER PROFESSIONS' COMPETENCIES AND CODES OF ETHICS

One of the ethical difficulties in professional interrelationships is that areas of competence and scope of practice differ (as do individual competencies within these broad categories). Refraining from giving colleagues work or teaching them activities which they are not qualified to provide is part of maintaining the ethical culture in mental health, as well. For example, the psychiatrists' code of ethics, with specific reference to psychologists, states that psychiatrists do not delegate any matter requiring the exercise of professional medical judgment. The psychologists' code indicates that psychologists do not promote the use of psychological assessment techniques by unqualified persons. In addition to the obligation to be aware of the special contributions of each of the mental health disciplines (which also allows one to make sensible referrals), there is the issue of awareness of the ethical codes by which they practice. Appendices A to E (pp. 193-317) contain the ethical codes of psychiatry, psychology, social work, marriage and family therapy, and counseling; the reader is encouraged to review them and note points of similarity and differences with his or her own profession's code.

Chapter 10

ETHICAL ISSUES IN RECORD KEEPING

Although there have been significant professional disagreements about the extent and desirability of record keeping, it has become clear that records in some form are essential to the responsible practice of the mental health professions. The mental health record serves several crucial functions: First, records are clinical tools, for example, reminding the clinician of important themes and perceptions related to the case, or providing information needed by colleagues who may subsequently become involved with the case. Second, records serve as legal documents in such circumstances as malpractice actions, divorce proceedings, or child custody cases. Third, insurance companies and other third parties rely on clinicians' records to document the amount, nature, and duration of services rendered.

Perhaps because of disputes about the extent of the need to keep records, the codified ethical standards of the various mental health professions offer little in the way of specific guidelines for record keeping (cf. *General Guidelines for Providers of Psychological Services,* American Psychological Association, 1987). This situation may be changing, however, as professionals have become increasingly aware of the ethical and legal implications of record keeping (American Psychiatric Association, 2001; NASW, 1999).

With or without specific standards, clinicians who practice responsibly must attend to a number of ethical concerns. Records can "speak" for the clinician or the patient: They can be used to document the provision of competent, responsible service; they can be used (or abused) to compromise the client's rights of confidentiality; and they can, when released to others, raise questions of patient's autonomy and informed consent. The importance of accurate records cannot be underestimated (Suisson, VandeCreek, & Knapp, 1987). Many ethical and competent therapists have been found negligent because they did not maintain adequate records. This chapter is devoted to the ethical dimensions of these and related issues raised in the course of record keeping. The first section suggests what might constitute relevant (and irrelevant) aspects of a client's chart. Second, we review some of the situations in which clinical information is released. Third, some general considerations in maintaining the security of records are described.

WHAT SHOULD BE INCLUDED IN RECORDS

A wide range of record-keeping practices exists among clinicians, ranging from avoidance of the practice to the keeping of almost verbatim accounts. At the one extreme, some clinicians contend that it is inappropriate to keep records at all. This position stems from one of two ideas: that record keeping (or at least note taking) disrupts the "here and now" nature of therapy or that record keeping (or rather the absence of records) provides protection against subpoena. At the other end of the spectrum are those clinicians who painstakingly record virtually every word the client says, making no effort to separate the important from the trivial. From an ethical perspective, both positions pose problems. Certainly without records or notes there is nothing to be released, but at the same time there is no way to document competent service or to remind yourself of concerns discussed with the client. On the other hand, while including everything in the chart obviously provides extensive documentation, it also increases the amount of client information that is revealed if the records are subpoenaed. It may even decrease the usefulness of the information to subsequent therapists, inasmuch as they may be reluctant to read a massive transcript.

In determining what should be included in charts, the clinician should consider his or her potential "audiences": to whom is the information being provided? Below are described the typical audiences for which the clinician writes, including the types of information that each audience requires.

1. *The clinician himself or herself, and other practitioners.* Records should be a resource to the clinician himself or herself. Patients come and go from treatment, and treatment is interrupted by illness, travel, and other external factors. It is unlikely that the clinician will have perfect recall of all relevant themes and issues important in treatment, which makes clinical notes necessary. In addition, patients move, need referrals to other practitioners with different specialties, or resume treatment with a different therapist after termination. These cases, too, require adequate records to serve the client properly. Indeed, the clinician should consider what information would prove useful if another clinician had to take over the case because of the initial therapist's sudden demise or incapacity. Further, if at some time in the future the client again seeks treatment, good records may make more efficient the subsequent assessment or treatment-planning process.

2. *The patient.* Patients themselves sometimes wish to review their charts (this issue is discussed in more detail later in this chapter) and typically have the right to do so. Although the clinical issues behind a request to review the record should be thoroughly explored, it is good clinical practice to write your notes in such a way that you would not be troubled unduly if the client himself or herself were to read them. Clients often are curious about what issues they discussed at earlier points in treatment, they sometimes suffer memory lapses about what "homework" the therapist assigned to them, and sometimes transference reactions generate suspicion about what the therapist is writing about them.

3. *Third-party payors.* Third-party payors routinely investigate what disorder is being treated to determine whether it is covered under the terms of the policy or contract. Insurance providers also want to know that services have actually been provided, and that the type of services provided are considered appropriate. The clinical record is a typical

means of documenting these factors. Although insurance carriers and, increasingly, managed care companies ask for very detailed, sensitive information, such information should not normally be volunteered, and the rationale for needing it should be questioned. For this reason, it is generally wise to keep financial records separate from clinical records in order to minimize the broadcasting of confidential information. A complete record, for insurance purposes, should not typically need to include more than date of service, type of service, charges and payments, plus the diagnosis of the disorder treated.

While not directly an ethical concern, an issue with ethical as well as legal implications is the increased attention that Medicare investigators are focusing on the documentation contained in practitioners' records. In some cases, charges of fraud are being brought against practitioners for failure to document that the services provided and billed for are "medically necessary" (Foxhall, 2000). Policies in this area are emerging and vary among localities, so we can offer no specific suggestions on this point except to suggest that the practitioner be aware of various rules and definitions, especially in determining what is medically necessary. Also, this trend reemphasizes the importance of documentation in general because it is generally considered by medical records professionals that "If it isn't documented, it didn't happen" (Foxhall, 2000, p. 51).

4. *The legal system* (courts and attorneys). As noted earlier, charts may be subpoenaed as part of court proceedings. Such actions include malpractice suits against the therapist, criminal actions against the client, or some form of civil action such as a divorce or custody suit. As a defense against a malpractice suit, it is important that records reflect that the clinician has been responsible in conceptualizing the case and devising a treatment plan. Issues of suicide risk and the potential for physical aggressiveness should be included (even if only to note that they have been ruled out) so that it is clear from the chart that these things have not simply been overlooked (Cohen, 1979). Also, if the client demonstrates any symptomatology that

may have a medical component, such as depression or thought disorder, the records should document that these factors have been considered, as well.

In summary, it is our recommendation that records be written with the potential audiences in mind, and that only information necessary to meet such needs be included in a client's chart. It is assumed that chart notes will be written in a professional, objective, and nonpejorative manner. It is critical that speculations be clearly defined as such and that caution be exercised in writing down allegations or hunches. Once something is included in a chart, it becomes archival and may be given more importance than it merits.

RELEASING RECORDS

There are a number of situations in which clinicians may be called upon to release their records or information contained in them. Below are listed the most common of these situations along with some of the ethical issues the clinician should consider.

Responding to Signed Releases of Information

There are numerous occasions on which the clinician is given permission by the client to release information. There are not necessarily any ethical problems with releasing information if the client has signed an appropriate release of information form (P. L. 104-191). However, certain factors in this process may have ethical implications. For one, it may be wise for the clinician to consider whether the client was able to give voluntary informed consent for the release. Kinzie, Holmes, and Arent (1985) surveyed 32 patients who released all or part of their psychiatric records; 81% of these patients felt that release of the information was mandatory in order to continue to receive medical, financial, or other help. This finding raises the question of whether releases of information are truly voluntary. If, for instance, refusing to sign a release of information form would result in an insurance company's refusal to pay the bill, then the client has been more or less coerced into giving permission to release information, regardless of fears about the risk to which he or she is exposed. While it should not be expected that the clinician absorb the loss if the client refuses to give permission to release information, the clinician should do whatever is possible to broaden the client's alternatives. The clinician may release only limited summaries (admittedly there is some cost to the therapist in preparing these separately from the clinical record), may attempt to change the third party's policy of demanding detailed information, or may discuss with the client (preferably in advance) the types of information that could be requested and who is likely to have access to that information. As we noted earlier, it is important to release no more than the information necessary for the purposes at hand. It is also important to note that the *clinician's* record-keeping policies are irrelevant to the insurance carrier's requests. That is, even if the practitioner keeps no records at all, the third-party payor may insist on detailed treatment information before authorizing payment. Discussion of the merits of continuing to deal with such a carrier and the possibilities for negotiation are unfortunately beyond the scope of this chapter.

If information is being released for legal purposes, the client should be informed that once permission is given, he or she is not usually able to restrict what is released. Clients involved in divorce actions, for instance, might understandably wish to release only that information which casts them in a positive light; they must be made aware that if they give permission to have information released for a certain purpose, all information that bears on that purpose is then accessible. A similar issue is found in disability insurance claims in which job stress is made an issue; the employee attempting to claim benefits may not be able to restrict the extent of information released.

Another issue the clinician must keep in mind when responding to a written release of information is that he or she is only empowered to release information about the person or persons who sign(s) the release (see also Chapter 4). For example, if a couple is seen in conjoint therapy and then at some later point the clinician receives a release of information form signed by only one of the partners, he or she is able only to release information about that one individual. The clinician would be wise to anticipate such an occurrence and keep charts in ways that would allow for the subsequent extraction of information on any individual client. Alternatively, the therapist might stipulate to the couple beforehand that records will be released only if both agree. If there is concern that a particularly litigious client will challenge such a policy, the practitioner should get a legal review of his or her informed consent statement.

A final point about responding to requests for releases of information relates to dealing with requests for information from other professionals. Good client care requires that a clinician seek information about a client's previous treatment. In fact, *Jablonski v. United States* (1983) held, in part, that a clinician was liable for not obtaining previous records. Thus for legal as well as ethical reasons, it is incumbent on responsible therapists to obtain prior records. Unfortunately, it is common to receive a very low rate of response to these requests. It bears mentioning here that it is extremely inconsiderate to fellow professionals (not to mention to your former patients) to ignore requests for records or information.

Responding to Subpoenas

Clinicians who are not familiar with the legal system can be intimidated when receiving a subpoena. As R. L. Schwitzgebel and R. K. Schwitzgebel (1980) have pointed out, however, there are different kinds of subpoenas, and not all of them demand the immediate release of records. Attorneys who have no legitimate right to the records will sometimes bluster and threaten, hoping that the clinician will be sufficiently intimidated to release the information. Clinicians who are not confident of their legal ground in this area or who have little familiarity with the subpoena process should get legal advice before turning over records. In addition, clients' attorneys should be consulted as well. As R. L. Schwitzgebel and R. K. Schwitzgebel (1980) have suggested, the best course of action when faced with a subpoena is to do nothing until one is sure of the appropriate course of action. Such a delay will not usually get a practitioner into trouble, but hasty and improper release of records might do so.

Allowing Clients Access to Their Own Records

The Federal Health Insurance Portability and Accountability Act of 1996 (HIPAA; P. L. 104-191) has reduced the clinician's discretion in deciding whether a client should have access to his or her own records. This Act states that, with certain exceptions, health care providers must permit an individual to inspect protected health information about the individual that the health care provider maintains. In addition, the individual has a right to receive a copy of this information. With the exception of "psycho-therapy notes" which have a specific definition, this requirement pertains both to mental health and medical records.

This Act is quite complicated; for clinicians, the most relevant *exceptions* to the requirement that clients have access to their own records are as follows:

1. An individual's access may be denied if the protected health information was obtained from someone other than a health care provider under a promise of confidentiality and the access requested would be reasonably likely to reveal the source of the information.
2. A licensed health care professional has determined, in the exercise of professional judgment, that the access requested is reasonably likely to endanger the life or physical safety of the individual or another person.
3. The protected health information makes reference to another person (unless the other person is a health care provider) and a licensed health care professional has determined, in the exercise of professional judgment, that the access requested is reasonably likely to cause substantial harm to the other person.
4. The request for access is made by the individual's personal representative, and a licensed health care professional has determined, in the exercise of professional judgment, that the provision of access to this representative is reasonably likely to cause substantial harm to the individual or another person.

In all cases but #1 above, the client should be provided with a right to review the denial.

As mentioned, a client in general does not have a right of access to psychotherapy *notes,* which are defined as notes recorded (in any medium) by a health care provider who is a mental health professional documenting or analyzing the contents of conversation during a private counseling session or a group, joint, or family counseling session and that are separated from the rest of the individual's medical record. This definition is not meant to include medication prescription and monitoring, session start and stop times, the modalities and frequencies of treatment furnished, results of clinical tests, and any summary of the following items: diagnosis, functional status, the treatment plan, symptoms, prognosis, and progress to date. Given these exceptions, it appears that the only thing that could be considered "psychotherapy notes" would be the practitioner's speculations and conjectures.

It is also important to note that HIPAA does not preempt state law if the state law is more stringent than these requirements.

Despite the limitations in the HIPAA legislation, practitioners still have some discretion in providing clients access to their charts. For example, it appears that clinicians have complete discretion in those parts of the record qualifying as psychotherapy notes. In addition, they have discretion determining what would endanger the life and safety of others.

From an ethical viewpoint, the question of whether to allow a client access to his or her records contains elements of the autonomy-paternalism conflict discussed earlier. If the clinician's decision were based solely on sustaining client autonomy, then the client would have total access to his or her records. If the decision were based completely on paternalism, then the client would justifiably be denied access to the records because the clinician would be empowered to act in the client's best interests, and client input would be unnecessary.

In light of our previous discussion of the autonomy-paternalism question, we believe that autonomy should be the overriding principle; clients should have access to information in their charts unless there is a justifiable reason to deny such access. The current revision of the Social Work *Code of Ethics* (NASW, 1999) is quite clear on this point. It states, "Social workers should limit clients' access to their records, or portions of their records, only in exceptional circumstances when there is compelling evidence that such access would cause serious harm to the client" (§ 1.08a).

While clients' requests to view their records are not common, the clinician would still be wise to anticipate such an eventuality. Records should be kept in a way that reflects solid professional judgment and respect for the client. Obviously, pejorative statements should be avoided.

GENERAL CONSIDERATIONS REGARDING
THE SECURING OF RECORDS

We assume that all practitioners are aware of their obligation to maintain their records in a way that protects the client's confidentiality. However, it is easy to get so accustomed to one's own routine that breaches of the confidentiality of records can occur in subtle and unexpected ways. Consider the illustration of a receptionist in a therapist's office who was discovered reading records of one of the clients, an attorney whom the receptionist was considering retaining. She was very open in explaining that she wanted to see whether the man could be trusted. She was a new receptionist, and the process of her training regarding the confidentiality of records was obviously lacking.

As another example, it is very easy to get into the habit of leaving client records on one's desk, making them accessible to other clients, office visitors, or cleaning staff. Such potential breaches are very numerous and, as noted, can occur even within the most responsible of record-keeping systems.

One area in which security of information is often compromised involves the telephone. Answering services should be carefully assessed to ensure that they understand proper procedure for taking and securing messages. Likewise, telephone machines should be carefully monitored, and care should be taken to ensure that no one but appropriate staff can hear incoming messages.

We recommend that practitioners periodically review their own behavior and their office practices with an eye toward such potential breaches. Clerical and other nonclinical staff should be included in this review; because nonclinical staff are not bound by the same ethical codes nor trained in appropriate procedures, careful orientation and supervision of them is necessary. Despite this difference in background, the practitioner bears the ultimate responsibility for the actions of his or her staff. Staff should be thoroughly trained in the relevant issues and reminded of their obligations to safeguard confidentiality. The practitioner might want to review and/or discuss record-keeping practices with a colleague in order to jointly benefit from fresh perspectives. An outsider may be able to point out things that the clinician, because of his or her familiarity with the routine, might not see.

Disposal of Records

For both practical and ethical reasons, the practitioner at some point may need to destroy records which are no longer relevant or useful. There are two important considerations in this regard: when to dispose of the records and how to do so. In terms of the first of these concerns, a number of factors need to be kept in mind. The practitioner needs to maintain records as long as there is a chance that they will be needed. As Koocher and Keith-Spiegel (1998) have pointed out, records may be needed for financial reasons (e.g., to serve as documentation for an IRS audit) or they may be needed to provide for continuity of care should a client again enter into treatment. Further, legal situations may arise which may make the details of treatment relevant at a later date.

Despite the obligation not to dispose of records prematurely, the length of time they should be kept is by no means clear. State and federal statutes vary as to the minimum length of time records should be kept. Koocher and Keith-Spiegel (1998) recommend keeping records at least 7 years from the termination of treatment, even if state statutes specify a shorter time period. This corresponds with the length of time that the IRS can audit a tax return. Psychologists are advised (American Psychological Association, 1993) to retain the full record for 3 years after completion of planned services or after the last date of contact with the consumer (whichever is later), and to maintain at least a summary of the record for an additional 12 years. The record may be entirely disposed of no sooner than 15 years after completion of planned services or after the date of the last contact, whichever is later. Special considerations apply when the client is a minor.

The practitioner may of course opt to keep records forever. Since relevant guidelines specify minimum time periods, such a course of action may be justified. However, this places other demands on the practitioner. Extremely old information may have become obsolete or irrelevant. Should this information be obtained by the legal system or employers, it may serve as the basis of inappropriate decisions. This concern places extra demands on the practitioner to secure records. Further, as will be discussed below, a practitioner who opts to keep records indefinitely should formulate plans for the disposition of the records in the event of death or severe disability.

As mentioned, in addition to the question of when to dispose of records, there is also the question of how to do so. It is important that they be disposed of in a safe, effective manner. Throwing confidential information in the trash is not adequate. A psychiatrist of our acquaintance was dismayed when he came to work one morning and found a draft of a psychiatric evaluation he had written lying on the sidewalk in front of his office door. He had thrown it in the garbage, the custodians had placed it in the dumpster, and the wind had blown it out. Any information with clients' names should be shredded (assuming that this will still allow the discharge of the ethical duty to recycle).

The psychologists' code of ethics mandates that psychologists must plan in advance so that the confidentiality of records is maintained regardless of whether the psychologist abruptly leaves the practice, moves, retires, becomes incapacitated, or dies (Koocher, 2004; McGee, 2004). Also, psychologists recognize that records and data must remain available to clients directly in some cases (e.g., custody evaluation reports). Because of a number of ethics complaints which involved withholding of records for nonpayment of fees, the psychologists' code explicitly prohibits linking these two activities. It is called "holding records hostage," and in the revised code it is now considered unethical.

The psychiatrists' code recognizes that the records must be "protected with extreme care" (American Psychiatric Association, 2001, § 4.1). No other guidance is given. The social workers' code of ethics states that "Social workers should transfer or dispose of clients' records in a manner that protects clients' confidentiality and is consistent with state statutes governing records and social work licensure" (NASW, 1999, § 1.07n). Marriage and family therapists are obligated to "store, safeguard, and dispose of client records in ways that maintain confidentiality and in accord with applicable laws and professional standards" (AAMFT, 2001, § 2.4). Counselors "are responsible for securing the safety and confidentiality of any counseling records they create, maintain, transfer, or destroy whether the records are written, taped, computerized, or stored in any other medium" (ACA, 1995, § B.4.b).

ELECTRONIC MEDICAL RECORDS

Over the next several years, we are likely to see a significant growth in the use of electronic medical records (EMR) in mental health as well as medical settings. There are a number of benefits to these records, including reducing storage space requirements, increasing access to records across settings, combining medical with billing records, and allowing for the integration of clinical practice guidelines and other aids to professional practice (Tierney et al., 1995).

Along with the increased benefits of electronic medical records come a number of ethical concerns. Foremost among these is the threat to confidentiality inherent in an online system with multiple access points. There is also the possibility of tampering with electronic records and of systems failing. Grams and Moyer (1997) among others, highlight the expanded risk of liability posed by the EMR. A useful guideline would be for clinicians to be as careful with their electronic records as they are with their paper records (and vice versa).

Before a practitioner adopts any electronic medical records system, it is important for him or her to assess whether the various ethical and legal problems inherent in such systems have been dealt with. Grams and Moyer (1997) suggest a 10-point framework that may prove helpful in making such decisions. They suggest, for instance, that the EMR use electronic signatures so that the person making the entry can be identified, and that once the entry is made, it is locked in so that it cannot be modified.

The authors also suggest that the EMR contain the entire patient record and not be a composite of paper and digital information. There should also be some type of backup in case the system fails. We also suggest that the system clearly limit access and that it keep a record of who accesses a file.

In summary, certain ethical principles (e.g., quality of care, accountability, etc.) can be well served through adopting an electronic medical records system; the standards of care needed to protect clients from any hazards posed by electronic records must be carefully evaluated and eliminated if possible.

Chapter 11

BILLING, COLLECTING, AND OTHER
FINANCIAL MATTERS

Despite the helping nature of the mental health professions, it is not unethical for clinicians to want to profit financially in their practices, nor is it inherently unethical to desire a relatively high income. However, because the practitioner's economic survival and standard of living depend on payment from clients and third-party sources, decision making about financial issues can easily be influenced by less-than-purely-ethical motives. In a subtle way, financial considerations may lead the practitioner to make ethically unjustifiable decisions, perhaps even without awareness that money motivates them. Conversely, as mental health practice becomes more commercial, practitioners who would prefer not to think about the monetary aspects of what they do may inadvertently put themselves or their clients in difficult situations.

The purpose of this chapter is to point out some of the more commonly observed ethical problems connected with the financial aspects of clinical practice. Whenever possible, we discuss practical solutions to the problems raised. In so doing, we are attempting to help providers become more comfortable with the fact that they are indeed in business and are selling their services; we also hope to demonstrate that a clinician can practice at a high level ethically and still survive financially, or as the old phrase has it, "do good and still do well."

The present chapter first covers potential ethical problems in charging and collecting fees from clients. Then insurance-related matters are discussed.

BILLING AND COLLECTING FROM CLIENTS

There are a number of financial matters that a practitioner must consider in dealing with clients. Among these are providing information about financial matters, collecting on bad debts, and considering whether to exchange professional services for services or goods from clients. In the following sections, each of these will be discussed.

Providing Information about Financial Matters

Practitioners vary considerably in their approaches to fee setting and other financial issues related to their clients. Because of the intimate nature of the therapeutic relationship, many practitioners become extremely uncomfortable with the reality that they are being paid for their time, and thus avoid bringing up such "details." These diffident clinicians reveal (or ask for) the minimum information necessary ("Do you have insurance?") or delay discussing fees and financial policies until the last possible minute. Others do not deal directly with money matters but delegate these tasks to the office staff. Still other practitioners view financial issues as fundamental to clinical practice and make them a part of therapy. While some latitude in these matters can certainly be appropriate, it is important to remember that the client has a right to know what types of services will be offered, their approximate duration, and the expected costs (Hare-Mustin et al., 1979). It is also helpful to note that a substantial number of ethics complaints are generated by conflict over billing practices. Thus it is not only ethical but also sound business practice to provide appropriate information before exposing clients to financial obligations they may not understand or may not be able to meet. The psychiatrists' code of ethics obligates the psychiatrist to be explicit about the provisions of the contract. The psychologists' code mandates that psychologists reach an agreement with consumers or payors as early as possible regarding fees and billing arrangements. Marriage and family therapists "make financial arrangements with clients, third-party payors, and supervisees that are reasonably understandable and conform to accepted professional practices" (AAMFT,

2001, § 7). They do not charge excessive fees; they disclose their fees at the beginning of services; and they accurately represent the services provided. Social workers are obligated to set fees that are "fair, reasonable, and commensurate with the services performed. Consideration should be given to clients' ability to pay" (NASW, 1999, § 1.13a). Counselors "clearly explain to clients, prior to entering the counseling relationship, all financial arrangements related to professional services including the use of collection agencies or legal measures for nonpayment" (ACA, 1995, A.10.a).

The nature of the therapeutic relationship makes this process different from the negotiations that would precede remodeling a kitchen or buying a car; some clinicians do not provide sufficient financial information because they have not developed a way of doing so that fits well with the flow of therapy. A client typically comes in for therapy highly distressed and anxious to begin. Thus to start off with a detailed description of financial and other matters necessary for informed consent may seem clumsy and inappropriate. Nonetheless, the prospective client needs the financial facts, perhaps especially so if he or she is highly distressed and perhaps vulnerable to becoming dependent on the therapist. As discussed in Chapter 5, a written handout covering all necessary information may be given to the client before the session. The clinician may simply ask if the handout was read and if there were any questions, and then (assuming that the client is competent to make such decisions) the clinician may obtain a signature consenting to the conditions outlined before the session begins. The information should include provisions for what steps will be taken if fees are not paid.

Collecting on Bad Debts

Mental health practitioners have another limitation not shared with other professionals who charge and collect fees—their options in collecting on bad debts. Faustman (1982) has pointed out that even turning the name and address of a client over to a collection agency can be a breach of confidentiality and, as such, may be prohibited unless specific consent has been provided by the client. For this reason we recommend that before treatment begins, the client be informed how bad debts will be collected and be asked to give written permission to turn bad debts over to a collection agency or an attorney. If such permission is not given, the practitioner must decide whether to provide treatment under restricted conditions. If indeed an overdue account accumulates (frequently after the client leaves therapy), the debtor should be warned with sufficient time to pay the debt before a collection agency is contacted. In fact, Bennett et al. (1990) urge caution in the use of collection agencies and emphasize the need for practitioners to know in detail how the collection agency will function.

Cohen (1979) found that fee disputes served as a stimulus for numerous legal actions against psychologists. Clients who leave therapy dissatisfied may respond to aggressive fee collection attempts by instituting malpractice suits against their therapists. While this is more a prudence issue than specifically an ethical concern, it is something clinicians would be advised to consider when deciding what to do with bad debts.

For both ethical and practical reasons, it would seem that the best solution to collecting on bad debts would be not to allow them to develop in the first place. Faustman (1982) suggests the following:

1. Expect payment at the time of service.
2. Use charge cards, filling out receipts in ways that do not reveal the therapeutic nature of the service.
3. Negotiate extended payment plans with clients.

Trading Services or Goods

Patients' poverty or inability to afford services faces the clinician with several options: service can be provided free (meeting the ethical obligation of psychologists, social workers, and psychiatrists, to provide some service pro bono), a sliding fee scale can be established, or a barter arrangement can be worked out. The last may seem a creative solution to the problem of the client's inability to pay for therapy; barter or trade could involve either goods or services. The therapist could, for example, provide psychotherapy in exchange for plumbing work. However, such arrangements are almost universally seen as unacceptable, at least among psychologists (Haas et al., 1986; Hall & Hare-Mustin, 1983). Part of the reason for this is that such arrangements are likely to create a problematic dual relationship between the practitioner and the client. It is not difficult to anticipate some of the other problems that these practices would lead to, such as difficulties equating the value of the services offered or dissatisfaction with the service by one or the other party.

The practice of bartering or trading goods, rather than services, is not so clear-cut from an ethical perspective (Hall & Hare-Mustin, 1983) because it is theoretically possible to trade therapeutic services for artwork or other material items without creating the inherent dual relationship problems that occur with trading services. The social worker profession frowns on this practice, making the statement that "Social workers should explore and may participate in bartering only in very limited circumstances when it can be demonstrated that such arrangements are an accepted practice among professionals in the local community, considered to be essential for the provision of services, negotiated without coercion, and entered into at the client's initiative and with the client's informed consent" (NASW, 1999, § 1.13b). In general, the American Association for Marriage and Family Therapy (2001) is also critical of the practice of accepting goods and services from clients (and supervisees) in exchange for professional services. It specifies that bartering should only be conducted if "(a) the supervisee or client requests it, (b) the relationship is not exploitative, (c) the professional relationship is not distorted, and (d) a clear written contract is established" (§ 7.5).

At the very least, however, if a clinician is considering providing therapy in exchange for some object of value, there should be a fair way of assessing the market value of the object, and this value should be agreed upon in advance. However, the clinician is cautioned that while such arrangements may make clinical services accessible to more individuals, they may also complicate the nature of the relationship if one or the other party is dissatisfied with the value received (of course this issue is relevant when cash is used to pay for services also).

In summary, while it is not inherently unethical to engage in bartering goods or services, it appears to us that the wise or prudent practitioner should avoid it in most if not all cases. The standard for psychologists (American Psychological Association, 2002) is that "Barter is the acceptance of goods, services, or other nonmonetary remuneration from clients/patients in return for psychological services. Psychologists may barter only if (1) it is not clinically contraindicated, and (2) the resulting arrangement is not exploitative" (§ 6.05). Counselors (ACA, 1995) have a more detailed standard. Their *Code of Ethics and Standards of Practice* states, "Counselors may participate in bartering only if the relationship is not exploitative, if the client requests it, if a clear written contract is established, and if such arrangements are an accepted practice among professionals in the community" (§ A.10.c).

ISSUES RELATED TO THIRD-PARTY PAYORS

The practitioner's dependence on insurance companies can lead to a number of practices that are ethically ill advised. Some of the more troublesome are described as follows.

Billable Diagnoses ("Up-Coding" or "Down-Coding")

Insurance policies do not typically cover all diagnostic categories. Usually, if the client's only diagnosis is a V-Code (American Psychiatric Association, 2000), such as parent-child or marital problems, insurance policies will not cover the service. This fact, combined with the client's need for insurance coverage to help defray the costs of treatment, can lead to the practice of giving the client a "billable" diagnosis even if such a diagnosis is not the most accurate.

In justifying this behavior, a clinician could come up with a number of explanations that are apparently ethical. It could be asserted, for example, that this is the only way for a client to get the help that he or she desperately needs, making inaccurate diagnosis the lesser of two ethical evils. In response to this, it should be noted that a practitioner who takes such an action is appropriating another party's funds to achieve what he or she believes to be moral ends. In other words, the practitioner is trying to be ethical with someone else's money, in that the insurance company is being asked to pay for an intervention that it would not pay for if all the facts were known. As an alternative, if finances are a problem and the client does not have a reimbursable diagnosis, the clinician may wish to consider seeing the client on a sliding scale, an extended pay schedule, or even as part of the clinician's pro-bono work. The clinician also exposes himself or herself to significant liability if the client later becomes upset about the diagnosis. This is a serious issue: Certain diagnoses interfere with the ability to obtain life insurance, to obtain security clearances, and to get reinsurance later (they are then considered "preexisting conditions"). These issues are not simple, and aside from the issues of honesty and paternalism involved, there is an issue of short-term versus long-term benefit to the client. The best policy, as the cliché says, is honesty. Working to change the insurance regulations or the cultural stigma around "mental illness" is a long-range goal but the only ethical alternative.

From a "financial survival" perspective, the clinician can take certain steps to minimize the economic impact he or she might experience if an insurance company refuses to reimburse for treatment of an accurately diagnosed disorder. First, the clinician should not guarantee insurance coverage. It should be clear at the start that paying the bill is the responsibility of the client even if the therapist will actively participate in filling out insurance forms.

Such a stance may be resisted by clients who would prefer that the clinician bill the insurance company, wait until payment is made, and then bill the client for the difference. Alternatively, the clinician may try other strategies that would make his or her policy more palatable. Use of a credit card allows the client to pay a bill on a more leisurely schedule without making the therapist dependent on insurance coverage. Use of this option might decrease dependence on insurance while being responsive to clients' needs for more time in meeting their obligations. However, one also has an obligation not to induce a client into a treatment relationship which he or she cannot afford to continue through to its proper conclusions. Also, therapists should consider what their policy would be if in the midst of therapy the client suffered large financial reversal. An immediate referral to a lower cost provider might be countertherapeutic: reduced fees may be necessary, or perhaps an extended payment plan. However, use of any of these options may stimulate resentment (in either party) and must be carefully monitored.

Writing Off Copayments

Another insurance-related practice that has ethical implications involves writing off the client's share of the bill and accepting the insurance reimbursement as payment in full. Insurance companies typically pay a certain percentage (often 50%-80%) of the practitioner's customary fee, and expect the client to pay the remainder, or copayment (Goodstein, 1983). In the case of financial hardship, waiving the copayment could be of considerable benefit to the client without costing the insurance company any money because the clinician would absorb the loss. This could be considered an ethical step in certain cases. Insurance companies might consider this inappropriate, but, according to Goodstein, the *occasional* waiving of copayments in cases of financial hardship may not present problems. However, where waiving the copayment becomes a routine practice, it could be viewed as a change in the clinician's usual and customary fee, with insurance companies in effect paying 100% of the clinician's fee. Such a policy could be viewed as deceptive or even fraudulent by an insurance company. Therefore, routinely waiving the copayment would not be considered ethical.

Confidentiality in Making Claims

In order to have insurance companies reimburse for therapeutic services, the client must typically sign a release-of-information form that allows the clinician to provide necessary claim information to the insurance company. Such a practice is routine and typically presents no problem ethically. The practitioner should keep certain considerations in mind, however. First, the release form is usually specific in stating that permission is given to provide information necessary for processing the claim. The implication is that care should be taken to release only information necessary for that purpose. Second, it may be wise to have the client consider where the billing information is going to go. Although the clinician is obligated to deal with clinical information in a sensitive and confidential manner, there is no clear-cut similar obligation on insurance company personnel. Therapists should inform themselves of the degree to which insurance carriers share information on diagnoses and services used through the Medical Information Bureau (MIB), a central information bank. It may be helpful for clients to know that they can request copies of their MIB files, although this is a somewhat laborious process (Medical Information Bureau, 1993).

The potential for breaches of confidentiality becomes greater in companies which process their own insurance claims. It would even be possible for a client's claim to be processed by a coworker. The clinician should explore such possibilities with the client and should be flexible in working out alternative payment plans if the client opts not to use insurance.

Responsibility for Clients When Insurance Benefits End

As people who work in mental health centers and other publicly sponsored agencies are aware, private practitioners sometimes treat clients until the insurance benefits have been exhausted and then refer them to a public agency. It may also be the case that other clients are simply terminated and left to their own devices when their benefits are used up. Ethical practitioners bear a responsibility to their patients which extends beyond insurance benefits. This is not to say that they must, regardless of other considerations, continue seeing clients who can no longer pay. It does mean that at the very least they are obligated to do more than simply tell patients to call a public agency. The clinician might, for example, explore treatment options that would be appropriate given the nature of the client's problem, or give the client names of specific practitioners at the agency, or take the responsibility for making sure that the transfer is handled in a constructive manner, and (with appropriate permission) provide the receiving therapist with appropriate background information. Clinical issues related to the termination of treatment should be sensitively considered as well.

This is an appropriate context in which to discuss the issue of abandonment. Throughout this book at various junctures we have made reference to the therapist's responsibility to continue treatment and not abandon patients. But what specifically constitutes "abandonment"? VandeCreek, Knapp, and Herzog (1987) have noted that the concept of abandonment has been dealt with more frequently in medical than in psychotherapeutic practice; in the medical arena abandonment refers to the failure to treat or appropriately refer a patient who needs treatment when the provider knows or should have known that continued treatment is necessary. There is no obligation to treat clients who do not need treatment—indeed, in several codes there is an ethical obligation to end professional relationships that are of no benefit to clients. However, the therapist and client may differ about the need for continued treatment. When this issue results in disagreement, the therapist must try to make clear his or her reasons for suggesting termination or referral and the client's options for resuming treatment in the future. It is prudent to document this discussion.

Chapter 12

PUBLIC STATEMENTS:
ADVERTISING, MEDIA APPEARANCES,
AND WORKSHOPS

Mental health professionals' opinions and ideas are in demand from the public, and it may serve ethical ends to give clinicians more public exposure. For example, a newspaper column on mental health matters may serve an important prevention function in a community, and a call-in advice line may provide immediate, free help to those who would really benefit from it. However, in addition to the possible benefits, there are risks inherent in making public statements.

The mental health practitioner commonly makes public statements (distinct from those made in confidence to patients and colleagues) in several arenas. First, there are professional publications, typically reviewed by peers; second, there are announcements about oneself and one's services made to the public; third, there are requests from the public for advice and information made via the media; and fourth, there are statements made to the press or the media (press conferences, interviews, etc). Statements made in professional publications are covered by the general standards of scientific and professional writing, and more specifically by the editorial policies of individual journals. Thus, it is on the remaining arenas that the present chapter focuses.

For the present purposes, the issues will be divided into three topics: (a) Issues concerning the provision of information about oneself. These typically concern questions of honesty and responsibility. (b) Information concerning general topics in one's area of expertise. This typically raises issues of competence, in addition to those of honesty and responsibility. (c) Information requested by specific persons. This typically adds the issue of conflicts of loyalty to those of honesty, competence, and responsibility.

Certainly some of these public activities are optional and voluntary, but it is increasingly likely that the practitioner will at some point in his or her career be called upon to make public statements. Such statements have the potential for raising or lowering the public's faith in both the person who makes the statement and in the profession represented by that person. Thus there is great concern with such activities by ethics enforcement bodies. If the mental health professions are to retain and enhance their credibility in the public's eyes, statements made by members of those professions must be accurate, honest, useful, and not self-serving.

PUBLIC STATEMENTS ABOUT ONESELF

The unavoidable public statements most practitioners make involve telephone listings, professional business cards, and professional announcements as public statements about themselves. In addition, for many practitioners who conduct workshops or publish, there are publishers' announcements, advertisements of workshops, course listings in catalogs, and the like. These sorts of announcements raise two kinds of issues. First there is the issue of "truth in advertising." That is, statements made to the public about oneself and one's services must be designed so as not to mislead or give the wrong impression. There are many ways in which a practitioner can capitalize on the public's lack of information or can use misleading phrases to create a distorted impression. For instance, consider the following statement: "Dr. X did graduate work in clinical psychology at Bogus College and then received his doctorate from State University." One may assume that Dr. X's degree is in clinical psychology, when it could as easily be in anything else. Such a statement is phrased in such a way as to mislead the reader. The phrase "received his doctorate in medieval literature from State University" is much more forthright. Another example might be the use of the term "institute" on one's letterhead when one is the sole provider of services in independent practice. The notion that one is the director of an institute would tend to mislead the naive consumer into thinking that more resources and prestige are involved than exist in reality. It is more accurate to describe oneself as a solo practitioner if this is in fact the case. This same reasoning underlies the mandatory obligation on psychologists to avoid testimonials from current psychotherapy clients in advertising of services; testimonials are inherently biased and not a scientifically valid means of assessing the effectiveness of services. It can also be argued (as it has been by the Federal Trade Commission) that the public's right to know and the professional's right to free trade must be balanced against the risk of misleading the potential consumer of services. This is the reason that not all clients are prohibited from giving testimonials.

The ethics codes of some of the mental health disciplines speak specifically about the professional's responsibility to be accurate in public statements. Psychologists "do not knowingly make public statements that are false, deceptive, or fraudulent" (American Psychological Association, 2002, Standard 5.01a). Marriage and family counselors "exercise special care when making public their professional recommendations and opinions through testimony or other public statements" (AAMFT, 2001, Standard 3.13). The *Code of Ethics and Standards of Practice* of the American Counseling Association gives counselors quite a bit of leeway when it comes to advertising. It states, "There are no restrictions on advertising by counselors except those that can be specifically justified to protect the public from deceptive practices," deceptive practices being those practices that are "false, misleading, deceptive, or fraudulent" (ACA, 1995, § C.3.a). Social workers "should ensure that their representations to clients, agencies, and the public of professional qualifications, credentials, education, competence, affiliations, services provided, or results to be achieved are accurate" (NASW, 1999, § 4.06c).

Some ethics codes also make it clear that professionals bear some responsibility not only for their own public statements but for those that others make about them, as well. Psychologists "who engage others to create or place public statements that promote their professional practice, products, or activities retain professional responsibility for such statements" (American Psycho-

logical Association, 2002, Standard 5.02b). Marriage and family
therapists "correct, wherever possible, false, misleading, or inaccurate information and representations made by others concerning the therapist's qualifications, services, or products" (AAMFT,
2001, Standard 8.6). Counselors also "make reasonable efforts to
ensure that statements made by others about them or the profession of counseling are accurate" (ACA, 1995, § C.3.c). Social
workers "should claim only those relevant professional credentials they actually possess and take steps to correct any inaccuracies or misrepresentations of their credentials by others" (NASW,
1999, § 4.06.c).

Testimonials pose yet another problem. In some forms of
mental health service, testimonials are an accepted business practice (e.g., organizational consulting, personal growth workshops).
The difficulty with soliciting psychotherapy clients or ex-clients
for testimonial purposes is that this may be misleading because
the clients may represent a distorted sample of consumers. In
addition, obtaining such testimonials may exploit the dependency
and trust of the client. Thus, the psychologists' code specifies that
psychologists "do not solicit testimonials from current therapy
clients/patients or other persons who because of their particular
circumstances are vulnerable to undue influence" (American Psychological Association, 2002, § 5.05). Similar wording is found in
the social workers' code of ethics, which states, "Social workers
should not engage in solicitation of testimonial endorsements (including solicitation of consent to use a client's prior statement as
a testimonial endorsement) from current clients or from other people who, because of their particular circumstances, are vulnerable to undue influence" (NASW, 1999, § 4.07b).

Perhaps because of the medical tradition of "grand rounds"
teaching activities which involve the presentation of patients, only
the psychiatrists' code of ethics deals directly with the presentation of patients or former patients to a public gathering or the
news media. This is considered ethical only if the patient is fully
informed of the consequences and gives written consent.

Interestingly, the psychiatrists' code includes public statements
under the section devoted to physicians' responsibility to participate in activities contributing to an improved community, underscoring the potential benefits of public statements. Psychiatrists
are specifically prohibited from rendering opinions about indi-

viduals in the public eye unless the physician has actually examined that person and has been granted permission to release a statement. In a similar vein, the psychologists' code prohibits "diagnosis in absentia."

An additional issue raised by self-promotional public statements is that of responsibility. It is not uncommon for third parties to edit or produce statements about a practitioner. Despite this fact, it is the practitioner's responsibility to ensure that statements are accurate and not misleading. Thus to claim that the book publisher distorted one's qualifications in composing the advertising for a book is to ignore the ethical mandate that one is responsible for one's professional activities. In general, it is wise to obtain "review and revision rights" from third parties who are publishing such material. In addition, if there is doubt about the accuracy of one's statements, peer review or ethics committee consultation should be sought. An issue of recent vintage is the accuracy of statements made about the practitioner by managed care networks that include him or her on their panels (Stromberg, 1992).

PUBLIC STATEMENTS ABOUT GENERAL TOPICS

Consider the following example: A professional practitioner and researcher is asked to appear on a local television show to discuss her research on sex role differences. While the results of her research are interesting, they are fairly specific and have limited generalizability. The interviewer, however, repeatedly asks such questions as, "Yes, but don't you think men today are unable to handle women's changing roles?" or "Why are men so out of touch with their feelings?" The research that was conducted did not bear on these questions.

Not uncommonly, practitioners are asked to provide information to the public about general topics. These requests may take the form of interviews in print or on the air (via television or radio) and frequently focus on some topic agreed upon in advance. Here the issues are related to those noted before but are somewhat broader. That is, the practitioner must be scrupulously honest in what he or she says. It is all too easy, under pressure to say something clever or provocative, to overstep the bounds of fact or the bounds of one's competence. It is humbling (but ethically obligatory) to point out that one is not an expert on a topic that is in fact beyond one's competence. Inevitably, questioners or interviewers will touch on these topics and, in the interest of entertaining or stimulating their audience, may insist on an answer. It is hard to convey in written form the seductive pressures induced by an insistent interviewer accompanied by bright lights and television cameras. Mental health professionals often want to please and will continue to speak when they should have stopped. Nonetheless these pressures must be resisted by the ethically responsible practitioner. Preparation for such situations is better than reaction, and "rehearsals" with trusted peers may be effective.

PUBLIC STATEMENTS ABOUT SPECIFIC PROBLEMS

It is possible that when providing information about general topics, the practitioner can qualify his or her answers by noting that these are general issues that may not apply to all persons. Increasingly, however, practitioners are being asked to participate in live electronic media events which expose them to the questions by specific persons about specific problems. These include phone-in talk shows, self-help shows, advice columns, and Internet "chat with the expert" interactive question-and-answer formats. Such circumstances are quite risky for the ethically responsible practitioner. A fundamental problem concerns divided loyalties, because the practitioner is being asked to use the caller's problem as a means of education (or perhaps entertainment) for the other members of the audience. At the same time, the practitioner has an ethical obligation to help the caller. Providing help to a particular caller may be misleading to listeners who do not share the specifics of the person's circumstances. For example, a caller who requests help with marital problems may seem to have circumstances similar to those of another listener with marital problems, but there may in fact be major differences. One caller may be married to a sadistic psychopath while the other may be married to an individual who simply lacks communication skills. It is important that the practitioner handle his or her responses in a way that misleads neither person.

In addition, as in the cases noted previously, the pressures to overstep the boundaries of one's competence are quite substantial. This is not simply a result of the demand characteristics of the television or radio studio; it may also be a result of the caller providing limited information and time for extensive questioning being unavailable. It is usually not possible in such circumstances to take refuge in denials of responsibility; the fact that the producers of the show do not allow the practitioner enough time to adequately assess the caller's circumstances is not a valid defense against charges that the practitioner who gives a hasty and inadequate response is acting irresponsibly and unethically.

It is worthy of note that the American Psychological Association now includes a division of media psychology. There are peer support groups, consultation resources, and evolving standards in this area that would be of considerable help to the practitioner who is considering entering the public domain in such a fashion.

In addition, to counterbalance the ethical problems, we should be aware that there are ethical principles that might be well served by public media presentations from clinicians. For example, media input might allow those too inhibited or constrained to seek professional help directly to receive at least some beneficial professional opinion. The preventive aspects of media psychology may also make a contribution to the quality of life. Thus the ethically responsible practitioner should not automatically refuse invitations for media appearances as too ethically troublesome. If the opportunity to make an impact through this avenue is appealing, careful preparation and self-discipline will be important.

GUIDELINES

1. *You cannot avoid responsibility for public statements.* For example, the responsible professional cannot take refuge in the fact that journalists might misquote him or her or might misattribute the facts. Instead, the responsible professional insists on the opportunity to review, revise, or edit public statements if at all possible. Similarly, responsibility in broadcast media cannot be avoided by claiming that one was subjected to irresistible pressure to answer inappropriate questions. Instead, the responsible professional negotiates beforehand to ensure his or her ability to refuse to answer inappropriate questions. This may also include ensuring that a time delay is installed on the telephone used in call-in shows so that one has a chance to screen calls. A further implication of this guideline is that

not only must you have rights of review for statements made in your name or with your name attached, but also you should have some options to rectify possible misstatements. These options might include having retractions published, or having follow-up (and corrected) interviews broadcast. The highly conscientious clinician may even consider providing brief consultation or crisis intervention for troubled callers or readers.

2. *Don't overstep the boundaries of competence.* This means that practitioners must know what the boundaries of their competence *are*. It also means that practitioners must become skillful, perhaps by rehearsal, at reminding interviewers, callers, producers, and others that their competence is not boundless.

3. *Be aware of potential conflicts of interest.* This includes reminding producers, publishers, interviewers, or other fellow participants of one's obligations to clients and potential clients as well as to the "host" of the particular medium in which one appears.

4. *Don't exploit callers.* This means that even though people naively ask for advice about apparently silly or inconsequential troubles, the practitioner must resist the temptation to exploit or mock them in a subtle way.

5. *Don't be afraid to seek consultation.* With the increasing body of knowledge accumulating in the area of media psychology, it is crucial to use this accumulated experience in preparing for media appearances.

Chapter 13

TESTS AND ASSESSMENT DEVICES

A tremendous range of instruments purporting to measure mental status, neuropsychological functioning, personality make-up, marital communication, intellectual capacity, vocational interests, moral development, and the like is available to the modern mental health practitioner. Psychological tests can be extremely useful in resolving diagnostic questions and developing effective treatment strategies. They can also overcome clinician biases. However, testing can also be misused. Further, although testing is typically considered the domain of psychologists because of their expertise with various psychological tests, all mental health practitioners are likely to have to deal with the dilemmas that the proliferation of tests present. Whether psychologist or not, clinicians may have questions about their clients that some form of testing would answer, they may receive test results on their clients from other clinicians or clinics, or they may be asked by clients to arrange for evaluation to answer specific questions. For this reason, ethical issues related to testing are relevant to all practitioners, not just to psychologists. However, the unique role of psychologists with regard to testing makes certain ethical issues particularly relevant to them. To deal with these separate issues, this chapter will be divided into two sections. The first will cover those aspects of testing that are relevant to all practitioners, and the second will highlight those issues specifically of concern to psychologists.

GENERAL ISSUES IN TESTING

Because all clinicians are likely to be involved with assessment in some form, there are certain ethical considerations that must be kept in mind. Those to be discussed here include practicing within one's area of expertise, sharing assessment information with clients in appropriate ways, and computerized assessment.

Practicing Within One's Area of Expertise

With testing, as with any other area of clinical practice, it is important that practitioners know the "boundaries" of their competence. Several factors make assessment especially fertile ground for boundary crossing. First is the accessibility of testing material. Though vendors of psychological tests are required to restrict access to test materials to those with the appropriate credentials, in practice it is extremely difficult to limit such access. Clinicians (and even nonclinicians) can easily purchase tests that they are not qualified to administer or interpret. Because of this, the burden is on each practitioner to be aware of the standards of training and knowledge required to administer, score, and interpret tests used in practice.

A second important issue is that tests often seem easier to interpret than they really are. Frequently, interpretive reports of scale scores allow practitioners to think that they understand what a test means when in actuality they do not. The Minnesota Multiphasic Personality Inventory (MMPI; Hathaway & McKinley, 1948) and its revision (MMPI-2; Hathaway & McKinley, 1989) may be the most visible examples of this sort of problem. Practitioners who know the names of the various scales, as well as the mean and standard deviation of the scales, may feel qualified to interpret the test. However, such individuals are often blissfully unaware of several intricacies of the tests. For example, scale names and what they actually measure are often highly divergent, the patterns or profiles of elevations are typically much more significant than individual scale elevations, and the configuration of validity scales is of great importance in correct interpretation. Further, the circumstances under which the test was administered and the emotional and motivational state of the test taker can greatly influence results. Although the MMPI is a clear-cut example of such problems, it is by no means the only example. Difficulties encountered by patients wrongly diagnosed in this fashion or individuals made anxious or given inappropriate treatment based on incorrectly interpreted or scored tests are among the possible outcomes.

Illustrative of how the MMPI may be misinterpreted by untrained users is the case of the nurse who looked over a client's MMPI profile and commented on how passive-dependent the client was. When asked how she had come to this conclusion, she replied, "Look how high his Pd score is" (Pd is actually the abbreviation for "Psychopathic deviate," which in itself is a somewhat misleading label for the constellation of traits measured in this scale). As a further illustration, a social worker speculated that, based on MMPI results, it appeared that one of his clients was homosexual, until it was pointed out to him that he was using a female profile sheet, thus causing the Mf (Masculinity-Femininity) Scale to be inaccurate. This example highlights two facts which a competent administrator of the test should know—first, the fact that male and female profile forms exist, and second, the relationship (or lack thereof) between Mf scores and homosexuality.

The solutions to these problems are largely ones of individual responsibility, of practitioners bearing the responsibility to know the limits of their competence. Responsible clinicians should know the acceptable scope of practice of their own discipline as codified in the ethical principles of that discipline, in published standards, and in relevant licensing laws. If practitioners are confronted by assessment questions with which they are not qualified to deal, referral to or consultation with an appropriately qualified colleague is in order.

Sharing Assessment Results With Clients

Practitioners may encounter situations in which they are requested to share assessment results with clients, even if they themselves did not perform the assessment. For instance, there may be cases in which the client was referred to another professional for testing, but no feedback was given by the evaluator. Rather, the treating therapist has the responsibility to inform the client of the results. In presenting assessment information, there is a wide range of attitudes regarding what is appropriate (Berndt, 1983). Some clinicians believe that honesty is the ruling principle and, as a consequence, share all results with the client without "editing." Other therapists opt for a more paternalistic stance, contending that the client has no need to know certain information and that it is up to the professional to decide what results are beneficial to share with the client.

The requirements of HIPAA (Public Law 104-191) have reduced therapist discretion in sharing test results with a client, as it has in other areas of professional practice. In the past, the professional who was sharing results could decide to withhold information such as an evaluee's IQ score if he or she determined that it would be harmful to share it. Now, no such discretion exists, except under very limited circumstances. While the point could be argued, this change can be looked at as a step in the direction of favoring informed consent (embodied in the principle of autonomy) over the clinician's responsibility to protect client welfare (embodied in the principle of beneficence).

HIPAA, however, does not eliminate the professional's responsibility to promote client welfare by paying considerable attention to how test information is presented to the evaluee. If, for instance, the evaluee is given a copy of the test results, the professional should take the time to review the results with the client and explain any areas of confusion. Further, the person presenting the results should do so in a sensitive and therapeutic manner. For instance, "You seem to have difficulty maintaining stable relationships" and "You have borderline personality tendencies" may convey the same concept, but, the former may be more therapeutic (as well as more clinically accurate) than the latter.

Before sharing assessment information with the client, it is important to be sure that the circumstances of assessment are such that the clinician can ethically do so. For instance, if there is confusion regarding who the client is, as discussed in Chapter 8, then the practitioner should be certain that he or she is justified in sharing assessment information with the person. A clinician working in a correctional or other institutional setting, for example, does not necessarily have the same freedom in sharing assessment information with the client as does a clinician in a private practice setting. In the institution, assessment information usually "belongs" to the institution rather than to the individual.

To summarize, when a practitioner is asked to share testing information with a client, the following questions should be considered:

1. Does the practitioner have the right to divulge the information, or does the information "belong" to someone else?
2. Will knowledge of the information be harmful to the client?
3. Is there any reason to withhold any part of the testing results?
4. Is it necessary to "translate" or revise the wording of the report to make the information understandable and/or useful to the client?

Computerized Assessment

The dramatic surge in the availability of computerized test administration, scoring, and interpretation services has increased the amount of assessment information available to clinicians. However, a number of ethical problems and concerns have accompanied this development (Matarazzo, 1986; Ryabik, Olson, & Kleim, 1984). Virtually every practitioner—psychologist or not—may be able to buy a computer disk that generates testing interpretations which, at least in surface appearance, seem similar to the psychological evaluations that a psychologist would provide. Such computerized scoring and interpretation services have proliferated dramatically in recent years. As mentioned, many test vendors have tight restrictions on whom they will sell tests to, but once the test is sold to a qualified individual, it is up to that individual to maintain test security. We suspect that the extent to which this security is maintained varies dramatically among individuals, especially when tests are bought for use by large clinics or agencies.

Although it may seem that trying to impose limitations on such resources reflects nothing more than professional territoriality, there are some very practical reasons to follow guidelines in using computerized assessment and interpretation. Specifically, while the output of computer programs can look very impressive, this output is based on tests developed by and interpreted by individual human beings. The chosen tests must have demonstrated reliability and validity for use in a particular setting with a particular client. The test scoring and interpretation must be accurate, valid, and appropriate. In sum, testing programs are no better than the humans behind them although the tests give the impression of being comparable to objective physical laboratory measurements in their precision and apparent completeness. Using such reports without awareness of the facts can lead to difficulty as easily as can misuse of the test itself.

It is also important to note that when psychologists conduct psychological evaluations they use more than one source of assessment information and that the evaluation reflects the synthesis of these sources so as to compensate for the error introduced by single measures used alone. A computerized test interpretation may look similar to a psychological evaluation, but it will be based on only one instrument and may be less accurate (Groth-Marnat, 1984). Further, a psychologist who conducts a psychological evaluation will have face-to-face contact with the test taker and will be able to consider the specific characteristics of the individual and the context in which the test is administered; this is not the case with computerized testing.

Standard 9.09c of the *Ethical Principles of Psychologists and Code of Conduct* (American Psychological Association, 2002) covers the issue of test scoring and interpretation services. Included in this section is the statement that "Psychologists retain responsibility for the appropriate application, interpretation, and use of assessment instruments, whether they score and interpret such tests themselves or use automated or other services." The *Code of Ethics and Standards of Practice* of the American Counseling Association (ACA, 1995) contains a similar statement which applies to counselors (§ E.2.b). Beyond these ethical standards, the American Psychological Association (1986) and the American Association of State Psychology Boards (1985) have developed guidelines for computer-based assessment and interpretation that should be read by anyone using such resources. Among other things, these guidelines specify that practitioners should only purchase and use computerized assessment programs that have demonstrated reliability and validity in the computerized form, that computerized assessments should only be conducted under circumstances similar to the ones in which they were validated, that the practitioner should use computer-generated reports only in the context of professional judgment and direct contact with the test taker, and that material from computer-generated interpretations should be identified as such.

ISSUES OF SPECIFIC RELEVANCE TO PSYCHOLOGISTS

As noted, Standard 9 of the *Ethical Principles of Psychologists and Code of Conduct* (American Psychological Association, 2002) is devoted to ethical issues related to assessment techniques. In addition, the American Psychological Association, in cooperation with the American Educational Research Association and the National Council on Measurement in Education, has published *Standards for Educational and Psychological Testing* (American Educational Research Association et al., 1999). The American Counseling Association has devoted an entire section to evaluation, assessment, and interpretation (ACA, 1995, § E). The material presented here should not be substituted for these various documents, but rather should be used as a summary of relevant concepts.

Beyond the expectations described in the previous sections of this chapter, the role of the psychologist implies other responsibilities in the process of assessment. What follows is a summary listing of some of the ethical considerations a psychologist should keep in mind. The considerations will be listed as a series of questions that the psychologist should ask himself or herself. Although we will not guarantee that this list is exhaustive, our belief is that dealing satisfactorily with the questions below would provide a large measure of confidence in the ethical appropriateness of testing practices.

Test Selection, Administration, and Scoring

1. Do the tests selected have acceptable psychometric properties based on current information?
2. Are the selected tests appropriate for the intended use?
3. Are the selected tests appropriate for the intended population?
4. Is the examiner competent and qualified to administer and interpret the selected tests?

Welfare of the Test Taker

1. Has the test taker given informed consent regarding testing procedures and use of results?
2. Is the testing environment conducive to test taking and free of distractions?

Sharing of Test Results

1. Has an acceptable release of information been signed, or is there some reason that such a release is unnecessary?
2. Can the person(s) receiving results be trusted to use them responsibly and sensitively? What security is there to prevent further release of the information?
3. Is more information being released than is necessary?
4. Is care being taken to avoid inappropriate labeling of the test taker?
5. Will results be conveyed to the test taker (either by the psychologist who administered the testing or by someone else) in a responsible, sensitive manner? If there are negative emotional consequences, is there a plan for dealing with them therapeutically?

Safeguarding Testing Materials and Results

1. Are test materials secured to prevent access and use by unqualified individuals?
2. Are test results stored in such a way as to protect the test taker's rights of confidentiality? For instance, if results are in a computer file, is there adequate security?
3. Is there a system for eliminating obsolete test results from charts or files?
4. To the extent possible, have you separated *test data* (raw and scaled scores, client/patient responses, phychologists' notes, etc.) from *test material* (manuals, instruments, protocols, test questions, etc.)? This is important because the American Psychological Association ethics code (2002) allows test data to be released pursuant to an authorization (Section 9.04) but expects psychologists to maintain the integrity of test material (Section 9.11).

CONCLUDING COMMENTS

Tests and testing results can be an important source of clinical information and a potent source of conflict as well. Wright (1981) noted that disputes over psychological testing were the second most frequent causes of malpractice actions (after disputes regarding fees). While this is, strictly speaking, primarily a psychologist's problem, other professionals should be aware that their use of tests and test results is both an opportunity and a risk. Increasingly, professionals must realize that they cannot afford to ignore the ever-more-sophisticated arsenal of tests available to them. At the same time, professionals have a clear obligation to use valid tests in a careful, appropriate manner.

Chapter 14

FORENSIC MENTAL HEALTH:
PRACTITIONERS IN THE COURTROOM

Few mental health practitioners will be in practice very long before having some contact with the justice system. Often these experiences come through involvement in courtroom proceedings. For some, the court experience is eagerly anticipated and sought out. For others, the receipt of a subpoena or a call from an attorney engenders panic. We consider it important for mental health practitioners, even those who do not specialize in forensic work, to understand some of the issues, temptations, and pitfalls encountered in interfacing with the court system so that they may be ready for their "day in court."

The seductive power of the courtroom, and the subtle gratification of being called as an expert, can sometimes blind the mental health professional to the need for particular skills and particular frames of mind necessary to both serve the court system and "do justice" to the complexity and integrity of the psychological issues at stake.

Partly in response to this state of affairs, there is increasing interest in the field regarding the tactics and strategies of "expert witnessing" (e.g., Brodsky, 1991; Shapiro, 1990). Much of this advice focuses on the mechanics of testifying; there is at least a modicum of attention paid to the notion of preparing properly, recognizing the boundaries of competence, and so forth. Judging by the sorts of complaints which reach ethics committees and licensing boards, however, more professional attention needs to be addressed to the issues of competence and quality in psychological courtroom work.

Of course, most if not all of the other concepts discussed in this book have applications to the legal setting. The relevant concepts would particularly include confidentiality and privilege, competence, dual relationships, and loyalty conflicts. However, given the unique nature of the court system and the mental health practitioner's role within it, it seems appropriate to devote a chapter specifically to court issues and their ethical implications.

Much work has been done discussing the role of the forensic mental health professional and the ethical considerations implicit in this role (e.g., Appelbaum, 1990; Golding, 1990; Melton et al., 1987). It should be made clear that the field of forensics is a fairly well-developed subspecialty, at least in psychology and psychiatry. Thus, board certification is available in both forensic psychology and forensic psychiatry, there are training programs in these areas, and so forth. There are also abundant sets of professional guidelines for the forensic psychologist (e.g., Division of Psychology and Law, 1991). The present discussion should not substitute for detailed study if one wishes to specialize in forensic mental health work; nevertheless, in the recognition that nonspecialist clinicians may be called upon to provide testimony or otherwise make contact with the legal system, we offer some introductory concepts. Additional sources should be consulted and further training should be obtained if one desires to pursue this further.

The present chapter is intended as an overview of the ethical considerations specifically relevant to dealing with the courts and is intended for those practitioners not specializing in courtroom work. For clarity, we will deal separately with situations where one is in court with one's client and when one is dealing with nonclients. These issues are relevant to questions of competence, as discussed in Chapter 3. The key ethical dimension here is whether one is serving one's clients by offering forensic mental health services when one is not well acquainted with the legal arena.

Competence in this arena, at least in part, involves the ability to balance the competing interests of scientific objectivity and advocacy, to communicate with a primarily lay audience without trivializing or overgeneralizing findings, to maintain the general ethical obligations (beneficence, autonomy, nonmaleficence) of the mental health professions, and the ability to understand and implement the specifics of one's own ethical code.

TESTIFYING ABOUT ONE'S CLIENT

Practitioners may be called to testify in court either by their client or by the opposing side. Which side initiates the request (or order) is critically important in determining what the practitioner does. Each of these contexts will be discussed in turn.

Giving Testimony Requested by the Client

If the request comes from the client himself or herself, then worries about breaching privilege are minimal because privilege is the client's to waive. However, for self-protection, a signed release of information from the client would be advisable. The implications of testifying should be discussed with the client in advance, as well. For example, could cross-examination take you beyond the area in which the client wished you to testify? If the privilege is waived by requesting your testimony, does the client recognize that this normally waives it *entirely?*

In order to minimize confusion or misunderstanding, if the client has initially sought treatment because it was court ordered or under other circumstances which would likely lead to courtroom involvement, these and related issues should be discussed and resolved at the beginning of treatment, and the therapist's role clarified at the outset.

Clients should be aware that they cannot restrict you to testifying only about the good things that they do and that your testimony will be subject to cross-examination. While you can say that your testimony will be limited only to relevant information, relevance is a legal determination once you are in court. If the client's attorney does not object to a question raised in cross-examination or the judge orders you to answer a question over the attorney's objections, then you must do so even if you and the client consider it irrelevant.

As mentioned in the chapter on confidentiality, a particularly troubling situation is that in which a therapist has seen more than one family member, for instance in marriage or family counseling. If some individuals are willing to waive privilege and some not, then the therapist can only testify about those individuals who have given permission. Trying to extract information only about certain individuals seen in a system context can be very tricky. Resolving these problems and deciding what can and cannot be said should be a matter negotiated among the therapist, the parties involved, and their counsel, as well as possibly the judge.

Giving Testimony Requested by the Opposing Side

If one's client is involved in a legal proceeding and the opposing side seeks the testimony, then the first issue for the practitioner to consider is whether privilege can be breached. As mentioned previously (see Chapter 4), simply receiving a subpoena does not allow you to breach privilege. Practitioners should seek their own legal advice upon receiving a subpoena as well as consulting with the client and the client's attorney. In some cases, the client may freely waive privilege; the clinician's ethical responsibility, as above, is to ensure that this is done with full awareness of the potential consequences. In other cases, the nature of the judicial proceedings may motivate the court to breach the client's privilege or may represent an automatic waiver of privilege. Examples of such situations would include suspected child abuse or a situation in which the client has made his or her own mental state an issue in the judicial proceedings. However, even if it seems obvious to you that the situation involves an implicit waiver of privilege, this should still be legally determined. That is, you would be wise always to claim privilege and then be ordered by the court to breach it.

Regardless of how the practitioner finds himself or herself in court, once there, and once the practitioner's testimony is allowed, other ethical questions are likely to occur. For one thing, dual relationship issues will probably emerge. However the practitioner characterizes his or her relationship with the client in the treatment setting (e.g., as a doctor whose purpose is to heal, as a consultant in living), courtroom testimony raises other roles for the practitioner: as an advocate, as an objective and detached evaluator, or possibly even as an antagonist. This can lead to a number of potential ethical violations, including betrayal or abandonment of the client (or at least the perception thereof).

Further, the adversarial nature of the courtroom procedure complicates the practitioner's role, in that there is considerable demand to present only that information which furthers one side or the other (Shapiro, 1992). Such a practice would be unethical, because biased information would be presented under the guise of scientific objectivity and detachment.

The competent expert should also know what he or she has *not* done, as well as what he or she has done (Shapiro,1990). This question is likely to be brought out by opposing counsel in any case because the attempt to discredit the expert witness will involve the inadequacy of the assessment or evaluation. Shapiro, 1990 notes, "There is a constant temptation in forensic work to go beyond the limits of one's competence and to render opinions in areas in which either the psychologist has no particular training or the state of knowledge is so meager that opinions should not be rendered" (p. 746).

Based on the preceding issues, we recommend three steps that a practitioner should take in providing court testimony about a client. The first is a restatement of something emphasized throughout this book—that it is wise to anticipate the potential for court involvement and to plan accordingly. Second, be clear as to your role vis-à-vis the court—to yourself, to your client, and to the court itself. If you have been a therapist to an individual, it must be clear to everyone involved that you should not be seen as an unbiased evaluator. Third, we consider it inappropriate from an ethical perspective to withhold information from the court. However, this statement must be clarified. Given the way court testimony works, you will be asked to respond to specific questions, and it is ethically appropriate to answer these questions honestly, even if your answers hurt your client. However, you are under no obligation to share information that is not sought. It is up to the attorneys to elicit from you the information they want, and, even if you consider information germane, it is not appropriate for you to volunteer it.

COURTROOM ROLES WITH NONCLIENTS

There are many roles a clinician can play in the courtroom in addition to the one mentioned previously. Examples can include conducting child custody evaluations, testimony as an expert witness about areas in which one has particular expertise, and conducting specialized evaluations for the court (e.g., competency, diminished capacity, guilty but mentally ill).

Garb (1991) in a useful discussion of the expert witness' task, notes that an expert witness should be able to help a judge or jury make more accurate judgments. If an expert witness cannot make more valid judgments than a judge or jury, then it is unlikely that the expert will be able to help a judge or jury improve the accuracy of their judgments (p. 452).

As mentioned, if one is considering doing a lot of courtroom work or doing work of a highly technical nature, then this should be considered specialty work, and the standards of training and competence should be commensurate. Custody evaluations and the specialized types of evaluations noted previously are examples. However, as a function of their area of specialization, practitioners without specific forensic training may be called upon to testify as expert witnesses. Following are listed some of the common ethical considerations and pitfalls in this role.

Special Prerogatives of the Expert Witness

Once an individual is qualified by the court as an expert witness, he or she is given a status not accorded nonexpert witnesses (Golding, 1990). Specifically, an expert witness can testify as to opinions and inferences. If a nonexpert witness presents such inferences and speculations, these statements are disqualified. With this authority comes a greater ethical responsibility. The courtroom setting is very seductive and can provide fertile ground for an expert witness to "expound" on his or her opinions and go beyond what can be supported (Koocher & Keith-Spiegel, 1998). This temptation should, of course, be avoided.

The Expert Witness Role

Practitioners not accustomed to courtroom work may assume a role different from the one that is appropriate. As Weissman (1991) has stated, the expert witness is neither an advocate (the attorney's role), nor the trier of fact (the judge's role). One implication of this statement is that, although the expert witness can provide information, it is up to the judge to make the final decision.

Another implication of the preceding statement is that an expert witness is obligated to present information in as objective and detached a manner as possible. There are a number of reasons that an expert witness can feel considerable pressure to distort or slant the data, present only arguments that support one side, or go beyond what can competently be asserted. First, there may be the feeling that if one gives testimony supportive of the side that hired him or her, there will be more such business in the future (the "hired gun" phenomenon). Second, attorneys can be quite persuasive and seductive in eliciting the desired information and can "turn the expert witness' head" in very subtle ways. While this may be seen as cause for cynicism and "attorney bashing," it must be remembered that the basis of our legal system is that the attorney is an advocate for the client and must present the best case possible. Indeed attorneys are ethically obligated to advocate as best they can for their client's cause. Is the expert witness in court more like the attorney? It is interesting to note that the faith in the legal adversarial system requires that lawyers become aggressive, competitive, and technically oriented. It is nowhere near as clear what might be the appropriate stance for the expert witness.

Conflicts of Ethical Principles

Many practitioners are used to a clinical setting, in which principles of beneficence and nonmaleficence are paramount. The testimony of an expert witness can be extremely damaging to someone involved in the court proceedings (Appelbaum, 1990). To distort the truth or withhold information, even in the service of promoting good or avoiding harm, would be considered unethical. Because of this, Appelbaum (1990) has contended that ethical principles in the courtroom should be looked at as different from those in clinical settings.

Differences Between Legal and Mental Health Concepts

One of the important considerations in doing courtroom work concerns the difference between legal and mental health concepts, and it is important for the practitioner to be aware of these differences (Koocher & Keith-Spiegel, 1998). The ethical principle involved here is one of competence. That is, the expert witness should have an understanding of how mental health terms translate into legal terms as they are relevant to the matter at hand. For instance, it is important to be able to differentiate mental illness as defined by statute from what one's own clinical definition of mental illness is (e.g., as synonymous with psychosis).

In addition, the mental health professional in the courtroom needs to have the judgment to know what facts are missing and in

which areas his or her conclusions need to be tempered or qualified or limited. Garb (1991) notes that "Even when mental health
professionals cannot make moderately accurate predictions they
can still assist judges and juries. For example, they can describe
the appropriate empirical research and simply conclude that the
prediction task is difficult or they may be able to help select appropriate statistical decision rules" (p. 453).

The belief sometimes expressed by less-than-competent
practitioners that the adversarial legal system can "protect itself"
and screen out incompetence through courtroom procedures,
rules of evidence, expert qualifying processes, and the like is
erroneous. The ethical perspective on professional competence
leads us to consider practitioners' obligations, regardless of
whether the legal system has safeguards, to practice at the highest
level of competence and with the aim of minimizing potential
harm (nonmaleficence; Beauchamp & Childress, 2001).

PROBLEMS

The forensic practitioner is vulnerable to a number of problems which we list here in terms of the virtue that is lacking:

Lack of Fidelity

This is exemplified by the expert witness who changes his
position between the time of agreeing with the attorney to testify
and actually appearing in court. Another example might be the
therapist who works with a couple on resolving their marital stresses
and appears in court on behalf of only one member of the couple
to argue for custody.

Lack of Prudence

This difficulty might be illustrated by the case of a psychologist who uses obsolete test results.

Lack of Discretion

This might be illustrated by the psychologist who casually
diagnoses the member of a couple whom he has not seen in treatment as "obviously a borderline."

Lack of Integrity

This might be illustrated by the expert witness who attempts to reconstruct a conversation held in therapy 15 years earlier without benefit of notes.

Lack of Humility

This might be illustrated by the expert witness who claims on the witness stand he can invariably detect schizophrenia.

Judging by the abundance of complaints to ethics committees and licensing boards about the actions of clinicians in the courtroom, the demand characteristics of the forensic arena exert considerable pressure on even highly trained mental health specialists to abandon the standards of excellence they might espouse in less pressured environments. The pressures of being on the witness stand and the seductions of extravagantly compensated evaluations and testimony can lead to enormous temptations to be a "hired gun" for the side which obtains one's services. Nonetheless, the ethical forensic practitioner must prepare for and resist these pressures.

Chapter 15

SERVICES PROVIDED BY TELEPHONE, INTERNET, AND EMAIL

The penetration of mobile and computer-based communication technology into our everyday life is apparent to almost all mental health clinicians. Most clinicians in private practice have been asked at least once (and perhaps routinely) by their patients if the patients can email information to the clinician. Certainly most clinicians have had patients bring in material from the Internet to ask questions about. It is also (unfortunately) the rare clinician who has not had a session interrupted by a patient's cell phone ringing. Another reference point is the widespread use of computers in American society. Budman (2000) notes that more than 50% of adults used computers in their homes in the year 2000 compared to 30% in 1996. Hundreds of new households join the Internet every hour.

Along with the expanding personal use of technology has come the expansion of electronic media into mental health services. Over the past decade we have seen the evolution of time-and-distance altering technologies into such services as the following: "pay-per-minute" telephone therapy; counseling and psychotherapy provided by email; synchronous (simultaneous) and asynchronous (delayed) chat rooms for individual or group therapy and support; and video conferencing as a two-way therapy medium. These approaches and others (see, for example, Barak, 1999; and Budman, 2000) have raised both enthusiasm and concern (Heinlen et al., 2003; Ragusea & VandeCreek, 2003).

Reasons for enthusiasm about these new technologies include the possibility that they will expand access to those potential clients or patients who cannot easily reach a trained mental health clinician. Those who live in rural settings, those who are isolated because they are homebound or have child care responsibilities, and those who have immediate crises and cannot travel to a distant clinic are all potential populations for whom immediate availability of services is a clear benefit. In addition the reduction of barriers to seeking mental health services is a benefit: travel time and the potential embarrassment of being seen in a mental health office are eliminated with electronically mediated services. Distance barriers to obtaining the most expert service in a particular area can also be eliminated since all of these technologies operate across state and national boundaries. In addition communicating via technologies that seem to increase anonymity may allow discussion of previously self-censored material to emerge.

Despite the enthusiasm about benefits arising from these new technologies, there are a number of reasons for concern. Three emerge as prominent in recent writings and clinicians' experience with communication technology: threats to privacy, limitations on the information available in the interaction, and difficulties with consumer protection. Let us consider each of these in turn.

Threats to privacy are numerous and impossible to eliminate completely. Although it is certainly true, as Grohol (1999) notes, that privacy is difficult if not impossible to maintain in the non-electronic world, the remarkable ease of access to information provided by electronic communications is a very real threat that must be considered. Patients calling their therapists on cell phones or even cordless phones can be easily overheard by eavesdroppers. Patients who use email to communicate with their therapists leave a "silicon trail" across each server through which the email passes; patients who use the Internet to contact their therapists will have "cookies" deposited on their computers that identify the computer for ease of reaccess to the web page; and those who use video conferencing may have others eavesdropping in the home or the workplace where their terminal is located. For these and other reasons there is tremendous concern about invasion of privacy when using electronic communications (Silk & Yager, 2003).

A second area of concern is limitations to the interaction. With the exception of video conferencing, all electronic media eliminate visual cues to the interaction. Email, chat rooms, and web-based interactions (unless they use streaming audio) eliminate auditory cues. Although advocates of computer-based services applaud the increased openness which comes from typing into a silent computer screen, others (e.g., Nagy, 1987) have long been concerned about whether the richness of the face-to-face interaction is fatally compromised by the elimination of these other cues. Subtle evidence of deeper emotional issues or of the contextual meaning of the statement are lost by communicating only with text and sometimes lost even on the telephone. However, the telephone is less susceptible to these problems since auditory cues and paralanguage cues (Haas, Benedict, & Kobos, 1996) provide considerable depth to the clinician's understanding. Nonetheless, it is important to realize that something may be missing when a face-to-face interaction is not possible. In addition, there is the problem of therapist's attention being limited. In a less rich communication environment, and in the presence of potential distractions of which the client might not be aware, the therapist could easily become inattentive or preoccupied with other things going on in his or her own environment.

Finally, there is the problem of consumer protection. Although this is much more of a legal than an ethical problem, it is still of concern to the conscientious clinician. Telephone therapy and Internet or email therapy can certainly take place across state lines, and this raises questions of where the service is being delivered. It would be reasonable to assume that the service is being delivered in the location where the client is located, and this may not be the location in which the therapist is licensed. It may also be difficult for clients to ensure their therapists' qualifications in the same way they do when entering in a physical office and seeing diplomas, staff members, colleagues, and so on. Also, under the rubric of consumer protection is the concern for widely differing charges for the service. Recent reviews of online charges suggest that it can cost up to $200 for a 50-minute session for a computer-based service. There is also the ethical problem (raised by Reed, McGauthlin, & Miholland, 2000) that the existence of these computer services may be used as a deterrent to obtaining face-to-face services because they may be cheaper for an agency to provide.

PROVIDING ETHICAL ELECTRONIC SERVICES

What are the ethical issues that must be addressed in order to provide such services with confidence? First, the clinician must ensure that there is no better option for the client; informed consent here, as elsewhere, is vital. Does the potential patient recognize that the service may be in some ways inferior to traditional face-to-face psychotherapy or mental health service? Obviously when a traditional treatment relationship has been established, these technological additions might improve continuity of treatment when therapists or clients are unavailable because of vacation, illness, or other circumstances. However, when this is a new treatment relationship and perhaps the only avenue for treatment, concern about the patient's informed consent should be paramount. As with other approaches to informed consent, making clear to the individual what the actual costs and risks are and what the costs and risks of alternative approaches to treatment might be is essential.

Second, the ethical clinician has a duty to make sure that he or she is competent to use whatever medium is chosen. For example, if email is used, does the clinician understand the methods by which the Internet service provider stores email messages and how often messages are removed from the provider's server? Has the clinician thought through how records will be kept? It is all too easy, for example, to simply keep a verbatim record of the emails sent by the patient. These then become the record and are potentially discoverable in a legal proceeding. Has the therapist become comfortable focusing his or her attention and not being distracted during Internet or telephone sessions? If all these conditions are met, it is in some respects no different to provide services using technology than it is to provide "traditional" services. Indeed, as the ethics code task force of the American Psychological Association point out (Fisher & Fried, 2003), professional ethics do not change when technology enters into the picture.

Thus, the time-tested ethical principles of beneficence, autonomy, and nonmaleficence here too can guide the ethical mental health practitioner through a variety of apparently new dilemmas.

Chapter 16

CLINICAL RESEARCH IN REAL-LIFE PRACTICE

Why do we include a chapter (albeit a short one) on clinical research in an ethics primer for practitioners? The fundamental reason is that the mental health professions distinguish themselves from spiritual, religious, or charismatic self-improvement techniques by virtue of their grounding in scientific evidence. Clinicians belong to a professional culture that is committed to creating and evolving an empirical foundation for its work. Thus, implicitly or explicitly, mental health practitioners must have a perspective on the linkage between ethical practice and their approach to research activities. In all mental health professions' codes of ethics, it is stated or implied that advancing the sciences contributing to improved mental health is an ethical obligation of the practitioner. Social workers (NASW, 1999), for instance, "should promote and facilitate evaluation and research to contribute to the development of knowledge" (§ 5.02b). "Psychologists are committed to increasing scientific and professional knowledge of behavior and people's understanding of themselves and others" American Psychological Association, 2002, Preamble). Psychiatrists "shall continue to study, apply, and advance scientific knowledge" (American Psychiatric Association, 2001, § 5). In the pursuit of these goals, even practitioners who do not themselves conduct empirical studies may be called upon to cooperate in others' clinical research activities. It is likely that even the solo independent practitioner will have opportunities to participate in clinical research at one or more points in a career. In addition to serving to advance the field of mental health in general, such participation can be personally and professionally rewarding to the practitioner. It is important that practitioners outside the academic setting be involved in clinical research because, in the absence of such involvement, studies are likely to be artificial and unrealistic. This chapter briefly reviews the pros and cons of participating in such research and highlights some of the dilemmas inherent in the major ethical issue, which is protecting the welfare of one's patients while advancing the scientific progress of one's discipline.

PRIMARY ETHICAL ISSUES

The practitioner's involvement in clinical research involves three major ethical issues. First, there is the consideration of wise investment of time. Practitioners must decide what sort of research is likely to be meaningful to themselves and their patients. Second, one must minimize dual relationships. Involvement in clinical research can present a loyalty conflict between responding to the needs of patients versus responding to the requirements of the study. Third, involvement in clinical research highlights the ethical obligation to promote the well-being of one's patients and to provide them informed consent. For example, practitioners must carefully assess the protection of patient identities and the effectiveness of informed-consent procedures.

The Practitioner's Responsibility

Ethical practitioners must have the option to decline participation in clinical research if it appears that the investment of their time and their patients' time will not result in any meaningful benefits either to the patients or the field as a whole. This can be a difficult judgment to make, especially if one is not an expert in the proposed area of research. In such cases it is necessary to rely on the judgment of the principal investigator, although one cannot abandon responsibility for making this judgment in the final analysis. Second, one cannot remove one's patients' autonomy by enrolling them in a clinical study without their consent. The patients must be informed, especially if the study involves any changes in the treatment that they would ordinarily get. Third, the practitioner must ensure that opportunities are available for detecting and remedying any negative effects which may result from the research involvement. For example, if some of the practitioner's patients are assigned to a waiting list or a "placebo control" group, the practitioner must reserve the option of providing some sort of treatment to these patients should their distress increase. The primary investigator should bear significant responsibility for the preceding concerns. However, a practitioner whose clients are involved in the research must also bear the responsibility for the maintenance of ethical conduct and procedures. He or she should avoid passive acquiescence to questionable practices, even in dealing with senior investigators with impressive research and academic credentials. An issue that is troublesome for many practitioners involves informing patients about their assignment to treatment versus control groups. If there is true random assignment, it is probably not in the interests of scientific validity to inform the patients of this, because those who are assigned to placebo or control groups may well withdraw from the study and thus bias the sample. On the other hand, patients have the right to know that random assignment will take place and must be willing to be assigned to the "other" condition. In general, the ethical researcher informs patients that assignment will take place, but may reserve the right not to inform the patients of the nature of the group to which they are assigned. A preferable resolution of this problem is to offer as the alternative treatment the best available treatment that is known for the patient's condition.

GUIDELINES

Based on the preceding, the following guidelines may prove useful in deciding whether to participate in a research project.

1. *Is it a worthwhile project?* Will the project answer important, relevant questions? Will it answer questions of importance to practitioners or theorists?
2. *Has it passed through appropriate committees?* A university-sponsored project typically should have passed a human-subjects committee. If the practitioner is part of an agency, it might be appropriate for that agency to establish a committee to ensure that the rights of subjects

are protected. If there is no committee to protect subjects' rights, the clinician's responsibilities to do so are increased.

3. *Has the client given informed consent?* While the purpose of the research may need to be withheld from the client, the client should be fully apprised of any information that may pertain to his or her decision to participate.

4. *Is there potential harm to the client? Do the benefits outweigh the harm?* This is obviously a very subjective decision, but the clinician should be able to be sure that there is minimal harm to the client and that the potential benefits outweigh any possible harm.

5. *Have appropriate safeguards been put into place for the client?* In the event of harm to the client, there should be remedial measures in place. The client should be free to withdraw at any time and should be aware of this freedom.

Chapter 17

PROFESSIONAL RENEWAL:
AVOIDING "PRACTITIONER DECAY"

Mental health practice is both art and science. Although improvements in one's practice of the art of psychotherapy do not depend on keeping abreast of the literature, the scientific aspects of the mental health disciplines require that one be familiar with current knowledge (ironically known as "the state of the art"). The explosion of information available with regard to new methods of treatment, revised views of existing methods, and new findings concerning the sources and symptoms of psychopathology mean that mental health knowledge can be considered to have a relatively short "half-life." This concept is drawn from Dubin (1972), who estimated that the half-life of a doctoral degree in psychology (as a measure of competence) was 10 to 12 years. In other words, over a decade's time approximately half of one's original fund of knowledge becomes irrelevant or wrong. This is analogous to the term coined by Campbell and Stanley (1963), "instrument decay," which refers to the decrease over time in the quality of a measuring tool. Regardless of the analogy, the issue of professional obsolescence can only be dealt with by continuing efforts to stay abreast of developments in one's areas of practice. This is perhaps simply another way of underscoring the obligation to be competent. The added perspective is that "competence" is not a permanent state achieved when one obtains the necessary credentials, but rather a continuing process of improving and refining one's diagnostic and treatment skills. Described below are two general areas in which practitioner decay can be problematic—professional knowledge and professional judgment and balance. For each, some specific considerations and guidelines will be described. We conclude with clinicians' ethical obligation to attend to their own well-being.

PROFESSIONAL KNOWLEDGE

Practitioners have the obligation to stay abreast of current professional knowledge, and the ethics codes of psychiatry, social work, psychology, counseling, and marriage and family therapy all contain provisions to this effect. Although it may seem at times that the accepted body of professional knowledge in mental health fields grows at an imperceptibly slow rate, and that we are perpetually rediscovering the wheel, when one compares the practice of psychotherapy now with practices of even a decade ago, there are numerous areas in which professional knowledge, techniques, and responsibilities have changed. Such areas as legal and ethical issues, the role of biological factors in behavioral problems, the role of distorted cognitions, advancements in diagnosis and assessment techniques, appropriate use of hypnosis, and treatment of sexual dysfunction are among areas that have shown marked changes. Further, even more traditional techniques such as psychoanalysis and behavior modification have grown and evolved.

Although it is incumbent on the practitioner to stay current, the task of assessing whether one is actually up to date in a particular area of practice is often very difficult. A guideline that a practitioner may wish to use in this regard involves a practice attorneys sometimes employ in cross-examining an opposing expert witness. The witness is asked to identify the most significant works in a particular area of practice and to indicate which ones he or she has read. The practitioner who asks himself or herself these questions may be able to obtain an estimate of his or her level of knowledge in the area in question. It is our assumption that most practitioners earnestly desire to stay current in terms of professional developments and techniques. However, given the heavy service demands that most practitioners face and the emotional strain that practitioners encounter, it is understandable that the time and energy needed to stay current may be sacrificed. When a clinician has spent a long day dealing with emotionally distressed individuals, the last thing he or she may want to do when arriving at home is to peruse journals. Further, when one considers the loss to a clinician's income that results from attending a 2- or 3-day seminar, it may be very tempting for many private practitioners to stay in the office and work instead.

The need to stay current has been recognized by many licensing authorities, and many licensing boards have established continuing professional education requirements that must be met to maintain one's license or certification. In addition, in some states it is necessary to provide evidence of continuing education to obtain malpractice insurance. Typically, however, such standards are minimal in scope and do little to focus attention on the content areas necessary to ensure that a professional will stay current. Often these activities are chosen more for their attractive location than their contribution to improved state-of-the-art practice.

Regardless of whether one is in a situation in which continuing education is required, the professional must bear major responsibility for ensuring exposure to advances in professional practice and changes in professional responsibilities. Practitioners should subscribe to journals that are relevant to their practice and become familiar with the contents, they should join appropriate professional organizations, and they should subscribe to professional listserve groups. It would be expected, in this regard, that practitioners will have the ability to assess the quality of the articles they read so that their practice is not guided by erroneous findings. The importance of this requirement is highlighted by the presence of such currently controversial topics as multiple personalities, ritual abuse, and false memories. In areas such as these, there is a wide range of opinion, the debate can be extremely emotional, and the negative consequences to clients of misapplied or inaccurate knowledge can be significant. As a result, it is especially important for the practitioner to maintain knowledge of research methodology and be aware of potential sources of bias in the reporting of research. Because it is difficult to read articles in all relevant areas of practice, the practitioner may wish to have information presented in a digested or condensed version. "State-of-the-art" lectures at national conventions are helpful, as are the opinions of senior colleagues regarding which professional journals have merit. Digesting or abstracting services have also become more widely available, including the following:

1. *PsycSCAN* (several available with specialty emphasis). This is an abbreviated literature search tool which provides citations and abstracts, as well as addresses to write to authors for reprints. It is available through the American Psychological Association (202-336-5600) and is offered at a reduced price for Association members. The mailing address is 750 First Street NE, Washington, DC 20002-4242. Their website is www.apa.org

2. *The Harvard Medical School Mental Health Letter.* This periodical is typically devoted to a theme (a particular disorder or method of treatment), and also includes brief reports of current research. It is published by Harvard Medical School (800-829-5379). The mailing address is 74 Fenwood Road, Boston, MA 02115. The website is www.hms.harvard.edu/

3. *Clinician's Research Digest.* Another source of brief article summaries from the psychological, psychiatric, and social work literature. Available from American Psychological Association, 750 First Street NE, Washington, DC 20002-4242 (202-336-5600, www.apa.org).

However, it must be remembered that many of these sources present information in a form that is difficult to evaluate methodologically, and there is a wide range of work cited, from the trivial and inaccurate to the profound and essential. It is important for the practitioner to assess the accuracy and relevance of the information presented. One option for helping the practitioner stay current involves the increased accessibility of computerized databases which contain references and abstracts of thousands of articles. While these databases were once prohibitively expensive and available only to institutions, they are now available to individuals with computers and modems and are reasonably inexpensive or free. In a short period of time, a practitioner can enter key words and review relevant abstracts. The National Library of Medicine (www.nlm.nih.gov/) and its associated database, *PubMed,* are good examples.

The Internet has had a revolutionary impact on resources available to the practitioner. Not many years ago, the number of practitioners who obtained professional information online was quite small. Today, those who do not use the Internet to obtain at least some professional information probably are, or will soon be, in the minority.

The vast array of information available online has the potential for dramatically improving the quality of professional services that a practitioner can provide. In a relatively short period of time and without leaving home or office, the practitioner can read the latest research on a variety of different disorders. When compared to the time that it takes to drive to a library and do a comparable search, this added convenience and practicality should significantly improve professional knowledge and skill.

However, the abundance and availability of information on the Internet can also be deceptive. When a practitioner enters a term through an Internet search engine, there is no quality control for what is returned, and results may be biased or erroneous. It is incumbent on the practitioner to have enough perspective and enough awareness of the professional area and of the source of information that he or she is not inappropriately influenced by what may be inaccurate information. One way to deal with this potential is to place primary reliance on sites of known credibility. The professional organizations of all of the disciplines referred to in this book have websites with much useful information for practitioners: marriage and family therapy (www.aamft.org), social work (www.naswdc.org), psychiatry (www.psych.org), psychology (www.apa.org), and counseling (www.counseling.org). In addition, useful information is available from federal agencies concerned with mental health and substance abuse issues, including the National Institute for Mental Health (www.nimh.nih.gov), the National Institute of Drug Abuse (www.drugabuse.gov), and the Substance Abuse and Mental Health Services Administration (www.mentalhealth.org).

Another step practitioners can take is to balance information obtained from the Internet with that obtained from other sources, such as seminars, journals, and professional colleagues.

While there is effort being directed toward assessing the ethical issues involved with providing professional services over the Internet, we are aware of no current efforts focused on dealing with the ethical issues involved in obtaining professional information from the Internet. Nonetheless, the ethical mandates of the various professions to provide competent service and protect the well-being of the client adds, in our estimation, an ethical dimension to how the practitioner acquires professional information through the Internet.

As important as having such resources available is maintaining the motivation to use them on a regular basis. Individuals with good self-control may have naturally good habits, or they may set up standards for themselves (e.g., "I won't watch television until I have reviewed 10 abstracts"). The rest of us may have to compensate for our lack of self-control by setting up a structure that requires us to stay current. One good way to do so is to establish a relationship with training institutions to provide ongoing contact with students. While the practitioner is sharing his or her years of experience with the student, the student is providing the practitioner with information regarding current techniques, approaches, and so on. Practitioners may also be able to make arrangements to teach classes, either at a university, community college, or community school. Although the financial rewards are meager from such teaching, one's time is still compensated to a certain extent, and the value to the practitioner is the enhancement of his or her own knowledge. It is conventional wisdom that to learn best, one should teach, and this is particularly true in mental health practice because much of the work goes on without peer involvement. In addition, the practitioner may find it useful to participate in journal clubs, case conferences, or similar professional activities. Finally, the practitioner should maintain active involvement with appropriate professional organizations, and if time allows, commit himself or herself to some function within the organization. Doing this gives the practitioner exposure to professional developments that is hard to obtain by interacting only with a journal or a computer terminal, and at the same time offers the opportunity to influence the development of one's own profession.

PROFESSIONAL JUDGMENT AND PROFESSIONAL BALANCE

In addition to maintaining awareness of advances in the field, there is a second component necessary for the practitioner to provide effective services to patients. This second element involves the use of professional judgment in knowing when to use one's knowledge or techniques effectively. A key factor that may reduce the quality of professional judgment over time, and that needs to be considered in one's ongoing efforts to prevent professional decay, is burnout. A therapist who feels overwhelmed and stressed in dealing with clients may not only be uninterested in professional reading or attending professional meetings, but may also show higher levels of anger or blame toward clients; may attempt to terminate them prematurely; may not invest emotionally to the extent appropriate; or may, in some other unconscious way, act out the resentment that he or she feels at having the responsibility for patients' welfare. As Freudenberger (1982) and others have pointed out, mental health professionals are at high risk for "burning out" because of the large emotional commitment necessary and the frustratingly small visible gains from that investment. Mental health practitioners must operate in an environment of uncertain effects from their work, and one in which they are frequently not appreciated for their helpfulness.

A related process that can occur to practitioners over time involves a gradual decrease in attention they pay to other aspects of their own lives besides work and an inappropriate emphasis on therapeutic relationships to meet certain needs (this is further discussed in Chapter 6). For instance, a therapist whose social life is restricted, for whatever reason, may seek to meet needs for affiliation through contact with clients, and his or her professional judgment may reflect this need rather than the clients' best interests. All practitioners are susceptible to decrements in professional judgment brought on by such factors as burnout or "life imbalance," and all would be wise to take steps to monitor and prevent such processes.

A necessary first step is open and sincere self-monitoring of one's motivations. As alluded to previously in this book, humans are all capable of significant levels of self-deception, and our status as therapists does not make us any different. It is hoped, however, that therapists are more attuned to this risk than many other professionals and are open to self-exploration as well as to the feedback of others, even if such feedback is hard to take. Although practitioners' individual decisions about balancing work, social, recreational, and spiritual aspects of their lives are personal matters, the result has professional and ethical relevance when balance (or lack of it) affects clinical work.

In summary, therapists should include in responsible and ethical practice efforts to take care of their own needs; it is not a sign of selfishness if one does not devote every waking hour to client care. In fact, we hope that the present discussion has suggested how such self-interest might make one a more effective professional, as well as a happier one.

Appendices*

TABLE OF CONTENTS

---

* Although the ethics codes reprinted in this text were current at the time of publication, professional associations periodically revise their codes and also publish supplemental materials dealing with ethical issues. Readers might want to periodically browse their professional association's website to obtain the most up-to-date information on ethical issues affecting their profession. At the time of publication of this book, these were the appropriate links for each profession:

AAMFT:	www.aamft.org/resources/lrmplan/ethics/index-nm.asp
ACA:	www.counseling.org/resources/ethics.htm
AMA/American Psychiatric Association:	www.psych.org/psych_pract/ethics/ethics.cfm
American Psychological Association:	http://www.apa.org/ethics/
NASW:	www.socialworkers.org/pubs/code/code.asp

Appendix A

CODE OF ETHICS
American Association For
Marriage and Family Therapy (AAMFT)*

PREAMBLE

The Board of Directors of the American Association for Marriage and Family Therapy (AAMFT) hereby promulgates, pursuant to Article 2, Section 2.013 of the Association's Bylaws, the Revised AAMFT Code of Ethics, effective July 1, 2001.

The AAMFT strives to honor the public trust in marriage and family therapists by setting standards for ethical practice as described in this Code. The ethical standards define professional expectations and are enforced by the AAMFT Ethics Committee. The absence of an explicit reference to a specific behavior or situation in the Code does not mean that the behavior is ethical or unethical. The standards are not exhaustive. Marriage and family therapists who are uncertain about the ethics of a particular course of action are encouraged to seek counsel from consultants, attorneys, supervisors, colleagues, or other appropriate authorities.

Both law and ethics govern the practice of marriage and family therapy. When making decisions regarding professional behavior, marriage and family therapists must consider the AAMFT Code of Ethics and applicable laws and regulations. If the AAMFT Code of Ethics pre-

---

*Reprinted with permission of the American Association for Marriage and Family Therapy, from the *AAMFT Code of Ethics*. This revised code was effective July 1, 2001. Copyright © 2001 by the American Association for Marriage and Family Therapy. Permission conveyed through Copyright Clearance Center, Inc.

scribes a standard higher than that required by law, marriage and family therapists must meet the higher standard of the AAMFT Code of Ethics. Marriage and family therapists comply with the mandates of law, but make known their commitment to the AAMFT Code of Ethics and take steps to resolve the conflict in a responsible manner. The AAMFT supports legal mandates for reporting of alleged unethical conduct.

The AAMFT Code of Ethics is binding on Members of AAMFT in all membership categories, AAMFT-Approved Supervisors, and applicants for membership and the Approved Supervisor designation (hereafter, AAMFT Member). AAMFT members have an obligation to be familiar with the AAMFT Code of Ethics and its application to their professional services. Lack of awareness or misunderstanding of an ethical standard is not a defense to a charge of unethical conduct.

The process for filing, investigating, and resolving complaints of unethical conduct is described in the current Procedures for Handling Ethical Matters of the AAMFT Ethics Committee. Persons accused are considered innocent by the Ethics Committee until proven guilty, except as otherwise provided, and are entitled to due process. If an AAMFT Member resigns in anticipation of, or during the course of, an ethics investigation, the Ethics Committee will complete its investigation. Any publication of action taken by the Association will include the fact that the Member attempted to resign during the investigation.

PRINCIPLE I: RESPONSIBILITY TO CLIENTS

Marriage and family therapists advance the welfare of families and individuals. They respect the rights of those persons seeking their assistance, and make reasonable efforts to ensure that their services are used appropriately.

1.1　Marriage and family therapists provide professional assistance to persons without discrimination on the basis of race, age, ethnicity, socioeconomic status, disability, gender, health status, religion, national origin, or sexual orientation.

1.2　Marriage and family therapists obtain appropriate informed consent to therapy or related procedures as early as feasible in the therapeutic relationship, and use language that is reasonably understandable to clients. The content of informed consent may vary depending upon the client and treatment plan; however, informed consent generally necessitates that the client: (a) has the capacity to consent; (b) has been adequately informed of significant information concerning treatment processes and procedures; (c) has been adequately informed of potential risks and benefits of treatments for which generally recognized standards do not yet exist; (d) has freely and without undue influence expressed consent; and (e) has provided consent that is appropriately documented. When persons, due to age or mental status, are legally incapable of giving informed consent, marriage and family therapists obtain informed permission from a legally authorized person, if such substitute consent is legally permissible.

1.3   Marriage and family therapists are aware of their influential positions with respect to clients, and they avoid exploiting the trust and dependency of such persons. Therapists, therefore, make every effort to avoid conditions and multiple relationships with clients that could impair professional judgment or increase the risk of exploitation. Such relationships include, but are not limited to, business or close personal relationships with a client or the clients' immediate family. When the risk of impairment or exploitation exists due to conditions or multiple roles, therapists take appropriate precautions.

1.4   Sexual intimacy with clients is prohibited.

1.5   Sexual intimacy with former clients is likely to be harmful and is therefore prohibited for two years following the termination of therapy or last professional contact. In an effort to avoid exploiting the trust and dependency of clients, marriage and family therapists should not engage in sexual intimacy with former clients after the two years following termination or last professional contact. Should therapists engage in sexual intimacy with former clients following two years after termination or last professional contact, the burden shifts to the therapist to demonstrate that there has been no exploitation or injury to the former client or to the client's immediate family.

1.6   Marriage and family therapists comply with applicable laws regarding the reporting of alleged unethical conduct.

1.7   Marriage and family therapists do not use their professional relationships with clients to further their own interests.

1.8   Marriage and family therapists respect the rights of clients to make decisions and help them to understand the consequences of these decisions. Therapists clearly advise the clients that they have the responsibility to make decisions regarding relationships such as cohabitation, marriage, divorce, separation, reconciliation, custody, and visitation.

1.9   Marriage and family therapists continue therapeutic relationships only so long as it is reasonably clear that clients are benefiting from the relationship.

1.10   Marriage and family therapists assist persons in obtaining other therapeutic services if the therapist is unable or unwilling, for appropriate reasons, to provide professional help.

1.11   Marriage and family therapists do not abandon or neglect clients in treatment without making reasonable arrangements for the continuation of such treatment.

1.12   Marriage and family therapists obtain written informed consent from clients before videotaping, audio recording, or permitting third-party observation.

1.13   Marriage and family therapists, upon agreeing to provide services to a person or entity at the request of a third party, clarify, to the extent feasible and at the outset of the service, the nature of the relationship with each party and the limits of confidentiality.

PRINCIPLE II: CONFIDENTIALITY

Marriage and family therapists have unique confidentiality concerns because the client in a therapeutic relationship may be more than one person. Therapists respect and guard the confidences of each individual client.

2.1   Marriage and family therapists disclose to clients and other interested parties, as early as feasible in their professional contacts, the nature of confidentiality and possible limitations of the clients' right to confidentiality. Therapists review with clients the circumstances where confidential information may be requested and where disclosure of confidential information may be legally required. Circumstances may necessitate repeated disclosures.

2.2   Marriage and family therapists do not disclose client confidences except by written authorization or waiver, or where mandated or permitted by law. Verbal authorization will not be sufficient except in emergency situations, unless prohibited by law. When providing couple, family or group treatment, the therapist does not disclose information outside the treatment context without a written authorization from each individual competent to execute a waiver. In the context of couple, family or group treatment, the therapist may not reveal any individual's confidences to others in the client unit without the prior written permission of that individual.

2.3   Marriage and family therapists use client and/or clinical materials in teaching, writing, consulting, research, and public presentations only if a written waiver has been obtained in accordance with Subprinciple 2.2, or when appropriate steps have been taken to protect client identity and confidentiality.

2.4   Marriage and family therapists store, safeguard, and dispose of client records in ways that maintain confidentiality and in accord with applicable laws and professional standards.

2.5   Subsequent to the therapist moving from the area, closing the practice, or upon the death of the therapist, a marriage and family therapist arranges for the storage, transfer, or disposal of client records in ways that maintain confidentiality and safeguard the welfare of clients.

2.6   Marriage and family therapists, when consulting with colleagues or referral sources, do not share confidential information that could reasonably lead to the identification of a client, research participant, supervisee, or other person with whom they have a confidential relationship unless they have obtained the prior written consent of the client, research participant, supervisee, or other person with whom they have a confidential relationship. Information may be shared only to the extent necessary to achieve the purposes of the consultation.

Principle III: Professional Competence and Integrity

Marriage and family therapists maintain high standards of professional competence and integrity.

3.1   Marriage and family therapists pursue knowledge of new developments and maintain competence in marriage and family therapy through education, training, or supervised experience.

3.2   Marriage and family therapists maintain adequate knowledge of and adhere to applicable laws, ethics, and professional standards.

3.3   Marriage and family therapists seek appropriate professional assistance for their personal problems or conflicts that may impair work performance or clinical judgment.

3.4   Marriage and family therapists do not provide services that create a conflict of interest that may impair work performance or clinical judgment.

3.5   Marriage and family therapists, as presenters, teachers, supervisors, consultants and researchers, are dedicated to high standards of scholarship, present accurate information, and disclose potential conflicts of interest.

3.6   Marriage and family therapists maintain accurate and adequate clinical and financial records.

3.7   While developing new skills in specialty areas, marriage and family therapists take steps to ensure the competence of their work and to protect clients from possible harm. Marriage and family therapists practice in specialty areas new to them only after appropriate education, training, or supervised experience.

3.8   Marriage and family therapists do not engage in sexual or other forms of harassment of clients, students, trainees, supervisees, employees, colleagues, or research subjects.

3.9   Marriage and family therapists do not engage in the exploitation of clients, students, trainees, supervisees, employees, colleagues, or research subjects.

3.10 Marriage and family therapists do not give to or receive from clients (a) gifts of substantial value or (b) gifts that impair the integrity or efficacy of the therapeutic relationship.

3.11 Marriage and family therapists do not diagnose, treat, or advise on problems outside the recognized boundaries of their competencies.

3.12 Marriage and family therapists make efforts to prevent the distortion or misuse of their clinical and research findings.

3.13 Marriage and family therapists, because of their ability to influence and alter the lives of others, exercise special care when making public their professional recommendations and opinions through testimony or other public statements.

3.14 To avoid a conflict of interests, marriage and family therapists who treat minors or adults involved in custody or visitation actions may not also perform forensic evaluations for custody, residence, or visitation of the minor. The marriage and family therapist who treats the minor may provide the court or mental health professional performing the evaluation with information about the minor from the marriage and family therapist's perspective as a treating marriage and family therapist, so long as the marriage and family therapist does not violate confidentiality.

3.15 Marriage and family therapists are in violation of this Code and subject to termination of membership or other appropriate action if they: (a) are convicted of any felony; (b) are convicted of a misdemeanor related to their qualifications or functions; (c) engage in conduct which could lead to conviction of a felony, or a misdemeanor related to their qualifications or functions; (d) are expelled from or disciplined by other professional organizations; (e) have their licenses or certificates suspended or revoked or are otherwise disciplined by regulatory bodies; (f) continue to practice marriage and family therapy while no longer competent to do so because they are impaired by physical or mental causes or the abuse of alcohol or other substances; or (g) fail to cooperate with the Association at any point from the inception of an ethical complaint through the completion of all proceedings regarding that complaint.

PRINCIPLE IV: RESPONSIBILITY TO STUDENTS AND SUPERVISEES

Marriage and family therapists do not exploit the trust and dependency of students and supervisees.

4.1   Marriage and family therapists are aware of their influential positions with respect to students and supervisees, and they avoid exploiting the trust and dependency of such persons. Therapists, therefore, make every effort to avoid conditions and multiple relationships that could impair professional objectivity or increase the risk of exploitation. When the risk of impairment or exploitation exists due to conditions or multiple roles, therapists take appropriate precautions.

4.2   Marriage and family therapists do not provide therapy to current students or supervisees.

4.3   Marriage and family therapists do not engage in sexual intimacy with students or supervisees during the evaluative or training relationship between the therapist and student or supervisee. Should a supervisor engage in sexual activity with a former supervisee, the burden of proof shifts to the supervisor to demonstrate that there has been no exploitation or injury to the supervisee.

4.4   Marriage and family therapists do not permit students or supervisees to perform or to hold themselves out as competent to perform professional services beyond their training, level of experience, and competence.

4.5   Marriage and family therapists take reasonable measures to ensure that services provided by supervisees are professional.

4.6   Marriage and family therapists avoid accepting as supervisees or students those individuals with whom a prior or existing relationship could compromise the therapist's objectivity. When such situations cannot be avoided, therapists take appropriate precautions to maintain objectivity. Examples of such relationships include, but are not limited to, those individuals with whom the therapist has a current or prior sexual, close personal, immediate familial, or therapeutic relationship.

4.7 Marriage and family therapists do not disclose supervisee confidences except by written authorization or waiver, or when mandated or permitted by law. In educational or training settings where there are multiple supervisors, disclosures are permitted only to other professional colleagues, administrators, or employers who share responsibility for training of the supervisee. Verbal authorization will not be sufficient except in emergency situations, unless prohibited by law.

PRINCIPLE V: RESPONSIBILITY TO RESEARCH PARTICIPANTS

Investigators respect the dignity and protect the welfare of research participants, and are aware of applicable laws and regulations and professional standards governing the conduct of research.

5.1 Investigators are responsible for making careful examinations of ethical acceptability in planning studies. To the extent that services to research participants may be compromised by participation in research, investigators seek the ethical advice of qualified professionals not directly involved in the investigation and observe safeguards to protect the rights of research participants.

5.2 Investigators requesting participant involvement in research inform participants of the aspects of the research that might reasonably be expected to influence willingness to participate. Investigators are especially sensitive to the possibility of diminished consent when participants are also receiving clinical services, or have impairments which limit understanding and/or communication, or when participants are children.

5.3 Investigators respect each participant's freedom to decline participation in or to withdraw from a research study at any time. This obligation requires special thought and consideration when investigators or other members of the research team are in positions of authority or influence over participants. Marriage and family therapists, therefore, make every effort to avoid multiple relationships with research participants that could impair professional judgment or increase the risk of exploitation.

5.4   Information obtained about a research participant during the course of an investigation is confidential unless there is a waiver previously obtained in writing. When the possibility exists that others, including family members, may obtain access to such information, this possibility, together with the plan for protecting confidentiality, is explained as part of the procedure for obtaining informed consent.

PRINCIPLE VI: RESPONSIBILITY TO THE PROFESSION

Marriage and family therapists respect the rights and responsibilities of professional colleagues and participate in activities that advance the goals of the profession.

6.1   Marriage and family therapists remain accountable to the standards of the profession when acting as members or employees of organizations. If the mandates of an organization with which a marriage and family therapist is affiliated, through employment, contract or otherwise, conflict with the AAMFT Code of Ethics, marriage and family therapists make known to the organization their commitment to the AAMFT Code of Ethics and attempt to resolve the conflict in a way that allows the fullest adherence to the Code of Ethics.

6.2   Marriage and family therapists assign publication credit to those who have contributed to a publication in proportion to their contributions and in accordance with customary professional publication practices.

6.3   Marriage and family therapists do not accept or require authorship credit for a publication based on research from a student's program, unless the therapist made a substantial contribution beyond being a faculty advisor or research committee member. Coauthorship on a student thesis, dissertation, or project should be determined in accordance with principles of fairness and justice.

6.4   Marriage and family therapists who are the authors of books or other materials that are published or distributed do not plagiarize or fail to cite persons to whom credit for original ideas or work is due.

6.5 Marriage and family therapists who are the authors of books or other materials published or distributed by an organization take reasonable precautions to ensure that the organization promotes and advertises the materials accurately and factually.

6.6 Marriage and family therapists participate in activities that contribute to a better community and society, including devoting a portion of their professional activity to services for which there is little or no financial return.

6.7 Marriage and family therapists are concerned with developing laws and regulations pertaining to marriage and family therapy that serve the public interest, and with altering such laws and regulations that are not in the public interest.

6.8 Marriage and family therapists encourage public participation in the design and delivery of professional services and in the regulation of practitioners.

Principle VII: Financial Arrangements

Marriage and family therapists make financial arrangements with clients, third-party payors, and supervisees that are reasonably understandable and conform to accepted professional practices.

7.1 Marriage and family therapists do not offer or accept kickbacks, rebates, bonuses, or other remuneration for referrals; fee-for-service arrangements are not prohibited.

7.2 Prior to entering into the therapeutic or supervisory relationship, marriage and family therapists clearly disclose and explain to clients and supervisees: (a) all financial arrangements and fees related to professional services, including charges for canceled or missed appointments; (b) the use of collection agencies or legal measures for nonpayment; and (c) the procedure for obtaining payment from the client, to the extent allowed by law, if payment is denied by the third-party payor. Once services have begun, therapists provide reasonable notice of any changes in fees or other charges.

7.3 Marriage and family therapists give reasonable notice to clients with unpaid balances of their intent to seek collection by agency or legal recourse. When such action is taken, therapists will not disclose clinical information.

7.4   Marriage and family therapists represent facts truthfully to clients, third-party payors, and supervisees regarding services rendered.

7.5   Marriage and family therapists ordinarily refrain from accepting goods and services from clients in return for services rendered. Bartering for professional services may be conducted only if: (a) the supervisee or client requests it, (b) the relationship is not exploitative, (c) the professional relationship is not distorted, and (d) a clear written contract is established.

7.6   Marriage and family therapists may not withhold records under their immediate control that are requested and needed for a client's treatment solely because payment has not been received for past services, except as otherwise provided by law.

PRINCIPLE VIII: ADVERTISING

Marriage and family therapists engage in appropriate informational activities, including those that enable the public, referral sources, or others to choose professional services on an informed basis.

8.1   Marriage and family therapists accurately represent their competencies, education, training, and experience relevant to their practice of marriage and family therapy.

8.2   Marriage and family therapists ensure that advertisements and publications in any media (such as directories, announcements, business cards, newspapers, radio, television, Internet, and facsimiles) convey information that is necessary for the public to make an appropriate selection of professional services. Information could include: (a) office information, such as name, address, telephone number, credit card acceptability, fees, languages spoken, and office hours; (b) qualifying clinical degree (see subprinciple 8.5); (c) other earned degrees (see subprinciple 8.5) and state or provincial licensures and/or certifications; (d) AAMFT clinical member status; and (e) description of practice.

8.3   Marriage and family therapists do not use names that could mislead the public concerning the identity, responsibility, source, and status of those practicing under that name, and do not hold themselves out as being partners or associates of a firm if they are not.

8.4   Marriage and family therapists do not use any professional identification (such as a business card, office sign, letterhead, Internet, or telephone or association directory listing) if it includes a statement or claim that is false, fraudulent, misleading, or deceptive.

8.5   In representing their educational qualifications, marriage and family therapists list and claim as evidence only those earned degrees: (a) from institutions accredited by regional accreditation sources recognized by the United States Department of Education, (b) from institutions recognized by states or provinces that license or certify marriage and family therapists, or (c) from equivalent foreign institutions.

8.6   Marriage and family therapists correct, wherever possible, false, misleading, or inaccurate information and representations made by others concerning the therapist's qualifications, services, or products.

8.7   Marriage and family therapists make certain that the qualifications of their employees or supervisees are represented in a manner that is not false, misleading, or deceptive.

8.8   Marriage and family therapists do not represent themselves as providing specialized services unless they have the appropriate education, training, or supervised experience.

Appendix B

CODE OF ETHICS AND
STANDARDS OF PRACTICE
Adopted by CACD 1996
American Counseling Association (ACA)*

PREAMBLE

The American Counseling Association is an educational, scientific, and professional organization whose members are dedicated to the enhancement of human development throughout the life-span. Association members recognize diversity in our society and embrace a cross-cultural approach in support of the worth, dignity, potential, and uniqueness of each individual.

The specification of a code of ethics enables the association to clarify to current and future members, and to those served by members, the nature of the ethical responsibilities held in common by its members. As the code of ethics of the association, this document establishes principles that define the ethical behavior of association members. All members of the American Counseling Association are required to adhere to the Code of Ethics and the Standards of Practice. The Code of Ethics will serve as the basis for processing ethical complaints initiated against members of the association.

Section A: The Counseling Relationship

A.1. Client Welfare

a. Primary Responsibility. The primary responsibility of coun-
    selors is to respect the dignity and to promote the welfare of
    clients.

b. Positive Growth and Development. Counselors encourage
    client growth and development in ways that foster the clients'
    interest and welfare; counselors avoid fostering dependent
    counseling relationships.

c. Counseling Plans. Counselors and their clients work jointly in
    devising integrated, individual counseling plans that offer rea-
    sonable promise of success and are consistent with abilities and
    circumstances of clients. Counselors and clients regularly re-
    view counseling plans to ensure their continued viability and
    effectiveness, respecting clients' freedom of choice. (See A.3.b.)

d. Family Involvement. Counselors recognize that families are
    usually important in clients' lives and strive to enlist family
    understanding and involvement as a positive resource, when
    appropriate.

e. Career and Employment Needs. Counselors work with their cli-
    ents in considering employment in jobs and circumstances that
    are consistent with the clients' overall abilities, vocational limi-
    tations, physical restrictions, general temperament, interest and
    aptitude patterns, social skills, education, general qualifications,
    and other relevant characteristics and needs. Counselors neither
    place nor participate in placing clients in positions that will re-
    sult in damaging the interest and the welfare of clients, employ-
    ers, or the public.

A.2. Respecting Diversity

a. Nondiscrimination. Counselors do not condone or engage in
    discrimination based on age, color, culture, disability, ethnic
    group, gender, race, religion, sexual orientation, marital status,
    or socioeconomic status. (See C.5.a., C.5.b., and D.1.i.)

b. Respecting Differences. Counselors will actively attempt to un-
    derstand the diverse cultural backgrounds of the clients with
    whom they work. This includes, but is not limited to, learning
    how the counselor's own cultural/ethnic/racial identity impacts
    her or his values and beliefs about the counseling process. (See
    E.8. and F.2.i.)

A.3. Client Rights

    a. Disclosure to Clients. When counseling is initiated, and throughout the counseling process as necessary, counselors inform clients of the purposes, goals, techniques, procedures, limitations, potential risks, and benefits of services to be performed, and other pertinent information. Counselors take steps to ensure that clients understand the implications of diagnosis, the intended use of tests and reports, fees, and billing arrangements. Clients have the right to expect confidentiality and to be provided with an explanation of its limitations, including supervision and/or treatment team professionals; to obtain clear information about their case records; to participate in the ongoing counseling plans; and to refuse any recommended services and be advised of the consequences of such refusal. (See E.5.a. and G.2.)

    b. Freedom of Choice. Counselors offer clients the freedom to choose whether to enter into a counseling relationship and to determine which professional(s) will provide counseling. Restrictions that limit choices of clients are fully explained. (See A.1.c.)

    c. Inability to Give Consent. When counseling minors or persons unable to give voluntary informed consent, counselors act in these clients' best interests. (See B.3.)

A.4. Clients Served by Others

If a client is receiving services from another mental health professional, counselors, with client consent, inform the professional persons already involved and develop clear agreements to avoid confusion and conflict for the client. (See C.6.c.)

A.5. Personal Needs and Values

    a. Personal Needs. In the counseling relationship, counselors are aware of the intimacy and responsibilities inherent in the counseling relationship, maintain respect for clients, and avoid actions that seek to meet their personal needs at the expense of clients.

    b. Personal Values. Counselors are aware of their own values, attitudes, beliefs, and behaviors and how these apply in a diverse society, and avoid imposing their values on clients. (See C.5.a.)

A.6. Dual Relationships

    a. Avoid When Possible. Counselors are aware of their influential positions with respect to clients, and they avoid exploiting the trust and dependency of clients. Counselors make every effort to avoid dual relationships with clients that could impair professional judgment or increase the risk of harm to clients. (Examples of such relationships include, but are not limited to, familial, social, financial, business, or close personal relationships with clients.) When a dual relationship cannot be avoided, counselors take appropriate professional precautions such as informed consent, consultation, supervision, and documentation to ensure that judgment is not impaired and no exploitation occurs. (See F.1.b.)

    b. Superior/Subordinate Relationships. Counselors do not accept as clients superiors or subordinates with whom they have administrative, supervisory, or evaluative relationships.

A.7. Sexual Intimacies With Clients

    a. Current Clients. Counselors do not have any type of sexual intimacies with clients and do not counsel persons with whom they have had a sexual relationship.

    b. Former Clients. Counselors do not engage in sexual intimacies with former clients within a minimum of 2 years after terminating the counseling relationship. Counselors who engage in such relationship after 2 years following termination have the responsibility to examine and document thoroughly that such relations did not have an exploitative nature, based on factors such as duration of counseling, amount of time since counseling, termination circumstances, client's personal history and mental status, adverse impact on the client, and actions by the counselor suggesting a plan to initiate a sexual relationship with the client after termination.

A.8. Multiple Clients

When counselors agree to provide counseling services to two or more persons who have a relationship (such as husband and wife, or parents and children), counselors clarify at the outset which person or persons are clients and the nature of the relationships they will have with each involved person. If it becomes apparent that counselors may be called upon to perform potentially conflicting roles, they clarify, adjust, or withdraw from roles appropriately. (See B.2. and B.4.d.)

A.9. Group Work

    a. Screening. Counselors screen prospective group counseling/ therapy participants. To the extent possible, counselors select members whose needs and goals are compatible with goals of the group, who will not impede the group process, and whose well-being will not be jeopardized by the group experience.

    b. Protecting Clients. In a group setting, counselors take reasonable precautions to protect clients from physical or psychological trauma.

A.10. Fees and Bartering (See D.3.a. and D.3.b.)

    a. Advance Understanding. Counselors clearly explain to clients, prior to entering the counseling relationship, all financial arrangements related to professional services including the use of collection agencies or legal measures for nonpayment. (A.11.c.)

    b. Establishing Fees. In establishing fees for professional counseling services, counselors consider the financial status of clients and locality. In the event that the established fee structure is inappropriate for a client, assistance is provided in attempting to find comparable servies of acceptable cost. (See A.10.d., D.3.a., and D.3.b.)

    c. Bartering Discouraged. Counselors ordinarily refrain from accepting goods or services from clients in return for counseling services because such arrangements create inherent potential for conflicts, exploitation, and distortion of the professional relationship. Counselors may participate in bartering only if the relationship is not exploitative, if the client requests it, if a clear written contract is established, and if such arrangements are an accepted practice among professionals in the community. (See A.6.a.)

    d. Pro Bono Service. Counselors contribute to society by devoting a portion of their professional activity to services for which there is little or no financial return (pro bono).

A.11. Termination and Referral

    a. Abandonment Prohibited. Counselors do not abandon or neglect clients in counseling. Counselors assist in making appropriate arrangements for the continuation of treatment, when necessary, during interruptions such as vacations, and following termination.

    b. Inability to Assist Clients. If counselors determine an inability to be of professional assistance to clients, they avoid entering or immediately terminate a counseling relationship. Counselors are knowledgeable about referral resources and suggest appropriate alternatives. If clients decline the suggested referral, counselors should discontinue the relationship.

c. Appropriate Termination. Counselors terminate a counseling relationship, securing client agreement when possible, when it is reasonably clear that the client is no longer benefiting, when services are no longer required, when counseling no longer serves the client's needs or interests, when clients do not pay fees charged, or when agency or institution limits do not allow provision of further counseling services. (See A.10.b. and C.2.g.)

A.12. Computer Technology

a. Use of Computers. When computer applications are used in counseling services, counselors ensure that (1) the client is intellectually, emotionally, and physically capable of using the computer application; (2) the computer application is appropriate for the needs of the client; (3) the client understands the purpose and operation of the computer applications; and (4) a follow-up of client use of a computer application is provided to correct possible misconceptions, discover inappropriate use, and assess subsequent needs.

b. Explanation of Limitations. Counselors ensure that clients are provided information as a part of the counseling relationship that adequately explains the limitations of computer technology.

c. Access to Computer Applications. Counselors provide for equal access to computer applications in counseling services. (See A.2.a.)

SECTION B: CONFIDENTIALITY

B.1. Right to Privacy

a. Respect for Privacy. Counselors respect their clients right to privacy and avoid illegal and unwarranted disclosures of confidential information. (See A.3.a. and B.6.a.)

b. Client Waiver. The right to privacy may be waived by the client or his or her legally recognized representative.

c. Exceptions. The general requirement that counselors keep information confidential does not apply when disclosure is required to prevent clear and imminent danger to the client or others or when legal requirements demand that confidential information be revealed. Counselors consult with other professionals when in doubt as to the validity of an exception.

    d. Contagious, Fatal Diseases. A counselor who receives information confirming that a client has a disease commonly known to be both communicable and fatal is justified in disclosing information to an identifiable third party, who by his or her relationship with the client is at a high risk of contracting the disease. Prior to making a disclosure the counselor should ascertain that the client has not already informed the third party about his or her disease and that the client is not intending to inform the third party in the immediate future. (See B.1.c. and B.1.f.)

    e. Court-Ordered Disclosure. When court ordered to release confidential information without a client's permission, counselors request to the court that the disclosure not be required due to potential harm to the client or counseling relationship. (See B.1.c.)

    f. Minimal Disclosure. When circumstances require the disclosure of confidential information, only essential information is revealed. To the extent possible, clients are informed before confidential information is disclosed.

    g. Explanation of Limitations. When counseling is initiated and throughout the counseling process as necessary, counselors inform clients of the limitations of confidentiality and identify foreseeable situations in which confidentiality must be breached. (See G.2.a.)

    h. Subordinates. Counselors make every effort to ensure that privacy and confidentiality of clients are maintained by subordinates including employees, supervisees, clerical assistants, and volunteers. (See B.1.a.)

    i. Treatment Teams. If client treatment will involve a continued review by a treatment team, the client will be informed of the team's existence and composition.

B.2. Groups and Families

    a. Group Work. In group work, counselors clearly define confidentiality and the parameters for the specific group being entered, explain its importance, and discuss the difficulties related to confidentiality involved in group work. The fact that confidentiality cannot be guaranteed is clearly communicated to group members.

    b. Family Counseling. In family counseling, information about one family member cannot be disclosed to another member without permission. Counselors protect the privacy rights of each family member. (See A.8., B.3., and B.4.d.)

B.3. Minor or Incompetent Clients

When counseling clients who are minors or individuals who are unable to give voluntary, informed consent, parents or guardians may be included in the counseling process as appropriate. Counselors act in the best interests of clients and take measures to safeguard confidentiality. (See A.3.c.)

B.4. Records

a. Requirement of Records. Counselors maintain records necessary for rendering professional services to their clients and as required by laws, regulations, or agency or institution procedures.

b. Confidentiality of Records. Counselors are responsible for securing the safety and confidentiality of any counseling records they create, maintain, transfer, or destroy whether the records are written, taped, computerized, or stored in any other medium. (See B.1.a.)

c. Permission to Record or Observe. Counselors obtain permission from clients prior to electronically recording or observing sessions. (See A.3.a.)

d. Client Access. Counselors recognize that counseling records are kept for the benefit of clients, and therefore provide access to records and copies of records when requested by competent clients, unless the records contain information that may be misleading and detrimental to the client. In situations involving multiple clients, access to records is limited to those parts of records that do not include confidential information related to another client. (See A.8., B.1.a., and B.2.b.)

e. Disclosure or Transfer. Counselors obtain written permission from clients to disclose or transfer records to legitimate third parties unless exceptions to confidentiality exist as listed in Section B.1. Steps are taken to ensure that receivers of counseling records are sensitive to their confidential nature.

B.5. Research and Training

a. Data Disguise Required. Use of data derived from counseling relationships for purposes of training, research, or publication is confined to content that is disguised to ensure the anonymity of the individuals involved. (See B.1.g. and G.3.d.)

    b. Agreement for Identification. Identification of a client in a presentation or publication is permissible only when the client has reviewed the material and has agreed to its presentation or publication. (See G.3.d.)

B.6. Consultation

    a. Respect for Privacy. Information obtained in a consulting relationship is discussed for professional purposes only with persons clearly concerned with the case. Written and oral reports present data germane to the purposes of the consultation, and every effort is made to protect client identity and avoid undue invasion of privacy.

    b. Cooperating Agencies. Before sharing information, counselors make efforts to ensure that there are defined policies in other agencies serving the counselor's clients that effectively protect the confidentiality of information.

SECTION C: PROFESSIONAL RESPONSIBILITY

C.1. Standards Knowledge

Counselors have a responsibility to read, understand, and follow the Code of Ethics and the Standards of Practice.

C.2. Professional Competence

    a. Boundaries of Competence. Counselors practice only within the boundaries of their competence, based on their education, training, supervised experience, state and national professional credentials, and appropriate professional experience. Counselors will demonstrate a commitment to gain knowledge, personal awareness, sensitivity, and skills pertinent to working with a diverse client population.

    b. New Specialty Areas of Practice. Counselors practice in specialty areas new to them only after appropriate education, training, and supervised experience. While developing skills in new specialty areas, counselors take steps to ensure the competence of their work and to protect others from possible harm.

    c. Qualified for Employment. Counselors accept employment only for positions for which they are qualified by education, training, supervised experience, state and national professional credentials, and appropriate professional experience. Counselors hire for professional counseling positions only individuals who are qualified and competent.

d. Monitor Effectiveness. Counselors continually monitor their effectiveness as professionals and take steps to improve when necessary. Counselors in private practice take reasonable steps to seek out peer supervision to evaluate their efficacy as counselors.

e. Ethical Issues Consultation. Counselors take reasonable steps to consult with other counselors or related professionals when they have questions regarding their ethical obligations or professional practice. (See H.1.)

f. Continuing Education. Counselors recognize the need for continuing education to maintain a reasonable level of awareness of current scientific and professional information in their fields of activity. They take steps to maintain competence in the skills they use, are open to new procedures, and keep current with the diverse and/or special populations with whom they work.

g. Impairment. Counselors refrain from offering or accepting professional services when their physical, mental, or emotional problems are likely to harm a client or others. They are alert to the signs of impairment, seek assistance for problems, and, if necessary, limit, suspend, or terminate their professional responsibilities. (See A.11.c.)

C.3. Advertising and Soliciting Clients

a. Accurate Advertising. There are no restrictions on advertising by counselors except those that can be specifically justified to protect the public from deceptive practices. Counselors advertise or represent their services to the public by identifying their credentials in an accurate manner that is not false, misleading, deceptive, or fraudulent. Counselors may only advertise the highest degree earned which is in counseling or a closely related field from a college or university that was accredited when the degree was awarded by one of the regional accrediting bodies recognized by the Council on Postsecondary Accreditation.

b. Testimonials. Counselors who use testimonials do not solicit them from clients or other persons who, because of their particular circumstances, may be vulnerable to undue influence.

c. Statements by Others. Counselors make reasonable efforts to ensure that statements made by others about them or the profession of counseling are accurate.

d. Recruiting Through Employment. Counselors do not use their places of employment or institutional affiliation to recruit or gain clients, supervisees, or consultees for their private practices. (See C.5.e.)

e. Products and Training Advertisements. Counselors who develop products related to their profession or conduct workshops or training events ensure that the advertisements concerning these products or events are accurate and disclose adequate information for consumers to make informed choices.

f. Promoting to Those Served. Counselors do not use counseling, teaching, training, or supervisory relationships to promote their products or training events in a manner that is deceptive or would exert undue influence on individuals who may be vulnerable. Counselors may adopt textbooks they have authored for instruction purposes.

g. Professional Association Involvement. Counselors actively participate in local, state, and national associations that foster the development and improvement of counseling.

C.4. Credentials

a. Credentials Claimed. Counselors claim or imply only professional credentials possessed and are responsible for correcting any known misrepresentations of their credentials by others. Professional credentials include graduate degrees in counseling or closely related mental health fields, accreditation of graduate programs, national voluntary certifications, government-issued certifications or licenses, ACA professional membership, or any other credential that might indicate to the public specialized knowledge or expertise in counseling.

b. ACA Professional Membership. ACA professional members may announce to the public their membership status. Regular members may not announce their ACA membership in a manner that might imply they are credentialed counselors.

c. Credential Guidelines. Counselors follow the guidelines for use of credentials that have been established by the entities that issue the credentials.

d. Misrepresentation of Credentials. Counselors do not attribute more to their credentials than the credentials represent, and do not imply that other counselors are not qualified because they do not possess certain credentials.

e. Doctoral Degrees From Other Fields. Counselors who hold a master's degree in counseling or a closely related mental health field, but hold a doctoral degree from other than counseling or a closely related field, do not use the title "Dr." in their practices and do not announce to the public in relation to their practice or status as a counselor that they hold a doctorate.

C.5. Public Responsibility

a. Nondiscrimination. Counselors do not discriminate against clients, students, or supervisees in a manner that has a negative impact based on their age, color, culture, disability, ethnic group, gender, race, religion, sexual orientation, or socioeconomic status, or for any other reason. (See A.2.a.)

b. Sexual Harassment. Counselors do not engage in sexual harassment. Sexual harassment is defined as sexual solicitation, physical advances, or verbal or nonverbal conduct that is sexual in nature, that occurs in connection with professional activities or roles, and that either (1) is unwelcome, is offensive, or creates a hostile workplace environment, and counselors know or are told this; or (2) is sufficiently severe or intense to be perceived as harassment to a reasonable person in the context. Sexual harassment can consist of a single intense or severe act or multiple persistent or pervasive acts.

c. Reports to Third Parties. Counselors are accurate, honest, and unbiased in reporting their professional activities and judgments to appropriate third parties including courts, health insurance companies, those who are the recipients of evaluation reports, and others. (See B.1.g.)

d. Media Presentations. When counselors provide advice or comment by means of public lectures, demonstrations, radio or television programs, prerecorded tapes, printed articles, mailed material, or other media, they take reasonable precautions to ensure that (1) the statements are based on appropriate professional counseling literature and practice; (2) the statements are otherwise consistent with the Code of Ethics and the Standards of Practice; and (3) the recipients of the information are not encouraged to infer that a professional counseling relationship has been established. (See C.6.b.)

e. Unjustified Gains. Counselors do not use their professional positions to seek or receive unjustified personal gains, sexual favors, unfair advantage, or unearned goods or services. (See C.3.d.)

C.6. Responsibility to Other Professionals

a. Different Approaches. Counselors are respectful of approaches to professional counseling that differ from their own. Counselors know and take into account the traditions and practices of other professional groups with which they work.

b. Personal Public Statements. When making personal statements in a public context, counselors clarify that they are speaking from their personal perspectives and that they are not speaking on behalf of all counselors or the profession. (See C.5.d.)

c. Clients Served by Others. When counselors learn that their clients are in a professional relationship with another mental health professional, they request release from clients to inform the other professionals and strive to establish positive and collaborative professional relationships. (See A.4.)

SECTION D: RELATIONSHIPS WITH OTHER PROFESSIONALS

D.1. Relationships With Employers and Employees

a. Role Definition. Counselors define and describe for their employers and employees the parameters and levels of their professional roles.

b. Agreements. Counselors establish working agreements with supervisors, colleagues, and subordinates regarding counseling or clinical relationships, confidentiality, adherence to professional standards, distinction between public and private material, maintenance and dissemination of recorded information, work load, and accountability. Working agreements in each instance are specified and made known to those concerned.

c. Negative Conditions. Counselors alert their employers to conditions that may be potentially disruptive or damaging to the counselor's professional responsibilities or that may limit their effectiveness.

d. Evaluation. Counselors submit regularly to professional review and evaluation by their supervisor or the appropriate representative of the employer.

e. In-Service. Counselors are responsible for in-service development of self and staff.

f. Goals. Counselors inform their staff of goals and programs.

g. Practices. Counselors provide personnel and agency practices that respect and enhance the rights and welfare of each employee and recipient of agency services. Counselors strive to maintain the highest levels of professional services.

h. Personnel Selection and Assignment. Counselors select competent staff and assign responsibilities compatible with their skills and experiences.

i. Discrimination. Counselors, as either employers or employees, do not engage in or condone practices that are inhumane, illegal, or unjustifiable (such as considerations based on age, color, culture, disability, ethnic group, gender, race, religion, sexual orientation, or socioeconomic status) in hiring, promotion, or training. (See A.2.a. and C.5.b.)

j. Professional Conduct. Counselors have a responsibility both to clients and to the agency or institution within which services are performed to maintain high standards of professional conduct.

k. Exploitative Relationships. Counselors do not engage in exploitative relationships with individuals over whom they have supervisory, evaluative, or instructional control or authority.

l. Employer Policies. The acceptance of employment in an agency or institution implies that counselors are in agreement with its general policies and principles. Counselors strive to reach agreement with employers as to acceptable standards of conduct that allow for changes in institutional policy conducive to the growth and development of clients.

D.2. Consultation (See B.6.)

a. Consultation as an Option. Counselors may choose to consult with any other professionally competent persons about their clients. In choosing consultants, counselors avoid placing the consultant in a conflict of interest situation that would preclude the consultant being a proper party to the counselor's efforts to help the client. Should counselors be engaged in a work setting that compromises this consultation standard, they consult with other professionals whenever possible to consider justifiable alternatives.

b. Consultant Competency. Counselors are reasonably certain that they have or the organization represented has the necessary competencies and resources for giving the kind of consulting services needed and that appropriate referral resources are available.

c. Understanding With Clients. When providing consultation, counselors attempt to develop with their clients a clear understanding of problem definition, goals for change, and predicted consequences of interventions selected.

d. Consultant Goals. The consulting relationship is one in which client adaptability and growth toward self-direction are consistently encouraged and cultivated. (See A.1.b.)

D.3. Fees for Referral

    a. Accepting Fees From Agency Clients. Counselors refuse a private fee or other remuneration for rendering services to persons who are entitled to such services through the counselor's employing agency or institution. The policies of a particular agency may make explicit provisions for agency clients to receive counseling services from members of its staff in private practice. In such instances, the clients must be informed of other options open to them should they seek private counseling services. (See A.10.a., A.11.b., and C.3.d.)

    b. Referral Fees. Counselors do not accept a referral fee from other professionals.

D.4. Subcontractor Arrangements

When counselors work as subcontractors for counseling services for a third party, they have a duty to inform clients of the limitations of confidentiality that the organization may place on counselors in providing counseling services to clients. The limits of such confidentiality ordinarily are discussed as part of the intake session. (See B.1.e. and B.1.f.)

SECTION E: EVALUATION, ASSESSMENT, AND INTERPRETATION

E.1. General

    a. Appraisal Techniques. The primary purpose of educational and psychological assessment is to provide measures that are objective and interpretable in either comparative or absolute terms. Counselors recognize the need to interpret the statements in this section as applying to the whole range of appraisal techniques, including test and nontest data.

    b. Client Welfare. Counselors promote the welfare and best interests of the client in the development, publication, and utilization of educational and psychological assessment techniques. They do not misuse assessment results and interpretations and take reasonable steps to prevent others from misusing the information these techniques provide. They respect the client's right to know the results, the interpretations made, and the bases for their conclusions and recommendations.

E.2. Competence to Use and Interpret Tests

a. Limits of Competence. Counselors recognize the limits of their competence and perform only those testing and assessment services for which they have been trained. They are familiar with reliability, validity, related standardization, error of measurement, and proper application of any technique utilized. Counselors using computer-based test interpretations are trained in the construct being measured and the specific instrument being used prior to using this type of computer application. Counselors take reasonable measures to ensure the proper use of psychological assessment techniques by persons under their supervision.

b. Appropriate Use. Counselors are responsible for the appropriate application, scoring, interpretation, and use of assessment instruments, whether they score and interpret such tests themselves or use computerized or other services.

c. Decisions Based on Results. Counselors responsible for decisions involving individuals or policies that are based on assessment results have a thorough understanding of educational and psychological measurement, including validation criteria, test research, and guidelines for test development and use.

d. Accurate Information. Counselors provide accurate information and avoid false claims or misconceptions when making statements about assessment instruments or techniques. Special efforts are made to avoid unwarranted connotations of such terms as IQ and grade equivalent scores. (See C.5.c.)

E.3. Informed Consent

a. Explanation to Clients. Prior to assessment, counselors explain the nature and purposes of assessment and the specific use of results in language the client (or other legally authorized person on behalf of the client) can understand, unless an explicit exception to this right has been agreed upon in advance. Regardless of whether scoring and interpretation are completed by counselors, by assistants, or by computer or other outside services, counselors take reasonable steps to ensure that appropriate explanations are given to the client.

b. Recipients of Results. The examinee's welfare, explicit understanding, and prior agreement determine the recipients of test results. Counselors include accurate and appropriate interpretations with any release of individual or group test results. (See B.1.a. and C.5.c.)

E.4. Release of Information to Competent Professionals

  a. Misuse of Results. Counselors do not misuse assessment results, including test results, and interpretations, and take reasonable steps to prevent the misuse of such by others. (See C.5.c.)
  b. Release of Raw Data. Counselors ordinarily release data (e.g., protocols, counseling or interview notes, or questionnaires) in which the client is identified only with the consent of the client or the client's legal representative. Such data are usually released only to persons recognized by counselors as competent to interpret the data. (See B.1.a.)

E.5. Proper Diagnosis of Mental Disorders

  a. Proper Diagnosis. Counselors take special care to provide proper diagnosis of mental disorders. Assessment techniques (including personal interview) used to determine client care (e.g., locus of treatment, type of treatment, or recommended follow-up) are carefully selected and appropriately used. (See A.3.a. and C.5.c.)
  b. Cultural Sensitivity. Counselors recognize that culture affects the manner in which clients' problems are defined. Clients' socioeconomic and cultural experience is considered when diagnosing mental disorders.

E.6. Test Selection

  a. Appropriateness of Instruments. Counselors carefully consider the validity, reliability, psychometric limitations, and appropriateness of instruments when selecting tests for use in a given situation or with a particular client.
  b. Culturally Diverse Populations. Counselors are cautious when selecting tests for culturally diverse populations to avoid inappropriateness of testing that may be outside of socialized behavioral or cognitive patterns.

E.7. Conditions of Test Administration

  a. Administration Conditions. Counselors administer tests under the same conditions that were established in their standardization. When tests are not administered under standard conditions or when unusual behavior or irregularities occur during the testing session, those conditions are noted in interpretation, and the results may be designated as invalid or of questionable validity.

b. Computer Administration. Counselors are responsible for ensuring that administration programs function properly to provide clients with accurate results when a computer or other electronic methods are used for test administration. (See A.12.b.)

c. Unsupervised Test Taking. Counselors do not permit unsupervised or inadequately supervised use of tests or assessments unless the tests or assessments are designed, intended, and validated for self-administration and/or scoring.

d. Disclosure of Favorable Conditions. Prior to test administration, conditions that produce most favorable test results are made known to the examinee.

E.8. Diversity in Testing

Counselors are cautious in using assessment techniques, making evaluations, and interpreting the performance of populations not represented in the norm group on which an instrument was standardized. They recognize the effects of age, color, culture, disability, ethnic group, gender, race, religion, sexual orientation, and socioeconomic status on test administration and interpretation and place test results in proper perspective with other relevant factors. (See A.2.a.)

E.9. Test Scoring and Interpretation

a. Reporting Reservations. In reporting assessment results, counselors indicate any reservations that exist regarding validity or reliability because of the circumstances of the assessment or the inappropriateness of the norms for the person tested.

b. Research Instruments. Counselors exercise caution when interpreting the results of research instruments possessing insufficient technical data to support respondent results. The specific purposes for the use of such instruments are stated explicitly to the examinee.

c. Testing Services. Counselors who provide test scoring and test interpretation services to support the assessment process confirm the validity of such interpretations. They accurately describe the purpose, norms, validity, reliability, and applications of the procedures and any special qualifications applicable to their use. The public offering of an automated test interpretations service is considered a professional-to-professional consultation. The formal responsibility of the consultant is to the consultee, but the ultimate and overriding responsibility is to the client.

E.10. Test Security

Counselors maintain the integrity and security of tests and other assessment techniques consistent with legal and contractual obligations. Counselors do not appropriate, reproduce, or modify published tests or parts thereof without acknowledgment and permission from the publisher.

E.11. Obsolete Tests and Outdated Test Results

Counselors do not use data or test results that are obsolete or outdated for the current purpose. Counselors make every effort to prevent the misuse of obsolete measures and test data by others.

E.12. Test Construction

Counselors use established scientific procedures, relevant standards, and current professional knowledge for test design in the development, publication, and utilization of educational and psychological assessment techniques.

SECTION F: TEACHING, TRAINING, AND SUPERVISION

F.1. Counselor Educators and Trainers

a. Educators as Teachers and Practitioners. Counselors who are responsible for developing, implementing, and supervising educational programs are skilled as teachers and practitioners. They are knowledgeable regarding the ethical, legal, and regulatory aspects of the profession, are skilled in applying that knowledge, and make students and supervisees aware of their responsibilities. Counselors conduct counselor education and training programs in an ethical manner and serve as role models for professional behavior. Counselor educators should make an effort to infuse material related to human diversity into all courses and/or workshops that are designed to promote the development of professional counselors.

b. Relationship Boundaries With Students and Supervisees. Counselors clearly define and maintain ethical, professional, and social relationship boundaries with their students and supervisees. They are aware of the differential in power that exists and the student's or supervisee's possible incomprehension of that power differential. Counselors explain to students and supervisees the potential for the relationship to become exploitive.

c. Sexual Relationships. Counselors do not engage in sexual relationships with students or supervisees and do not subject them to sexual harassment. (See A.6. and C.5.b.)

d. Contributions to Research. Counselors give credit to students or supervisees for their contributions to research and scholarly projects. Credit is given through coauthorship, acknowledgment, footnote statement, or other appropriate means, in accordance with such contributions. (See G.4.b. and G.4.c.)

e. Close Relatives. Counselors do not accept close relatives as students or supervisees.

f. Supervision Preparation. Counselors who offer clinical supervision services are adequately prepared in supervision methods and techniques. Counselors who are doctoral students serving as practicum or internship supervisors to master's level students are adequately prepared and supervised by the training program.

g. Responsibility for Services to Clients. Counselors who supervise the counseling services of others take reasonable measures to ensure that counseling services provided to clients are professional.

h. Endorsement. Counselors do not endorse students or supervisees for certification, licensure, employment, or completion of an academic or training program if they believe students or supervisees are not qualified for the endorsement. Counselors take reasonable steps to assist students or supervisees who are not qualified for endorsement to become qualified.

F.2. Counselor Education and Training Programs

a. Orientation. Prior to admission, counselors orient prospective students to the counselor education or training program's expectations, including but not limited to the following: (1) the type and level of skill acquisition required for successful completion of the training, (2) subject matter to be covered, (3) basis for evaluation, (4) training components that encourage self-growth or self-disclosure as part of the training process, (5) the type of supervision settings and requirements of the sites for required clinical field experiences, (6) student and supervisee evaluation and dismissal policies and procedures, and (7) up-to-date employment prospects for graduates.

b. Integration of Study and Practice. Counselors establish counselor education and training programs that integrate academic study and supervised practice.

c. Evaluation. Counselors clearly state to students and supervisees, in advance of training, the levels of competency expected, appraisal methods, and timing of evaluations for both didactic and experiential components. Counselors provide students and supervisees with periodic performance appraisal and evaluation feedback throughout the training program.

d. Teaching Ethics. Counselors make students and supervisees aware of the ethical responsibilities and standards of the profession and the students' and supervisees' ethical responsibilities to the profession. (See C.1. and F.3.e.)

e. Peer Relationships. When students or supervisees are assigned to lead counseling groups or provide clinical supervision for their peers, counselors take steps to ensure that students and supervisees placed in these roles do not have personal or adverse relationships with peers and that they understand they have the same ethical obligations as counselor educators, trainers, and supervisors. Counselors make every effort to ensure that the rights of peers are not compromised when students or supervisees are assigned to lead counseling groups or provide clinical supervision.

f. Varied Theoretical Positions. Counselors present varied theoretical positions so that students and supervisees may make comparisons and have opportunities to develop their own positions. Counselors provide information concerning the scientific bases of professional practice. (See C.6.a.)

g. Field Placements. Counselors develop clear policies within their training program regarding field placement and other clinical experiences. Counselors provide clearly stated roles and responsibilities for the student or supervisee, the site supervisor, and the program supervisor. They confirm that site supervisors are qualified to provide supervision and are informed of their professional and ethical responsibilities in this role.

h. Dual Relationships as Supervisors. Counselors avoid dual relationships such as performing the role of site supervisor and training program supervisor in the student's or supervisee's training program. Counselors do not accept any form of professional services, fees, commissions, reimbursement, or remuneration from a site for student or supervisee placement.

i. Diversity in Programs. Counselors are responsive to their institution's and program's recruitment and retention needs for training program administrators, faculty, and students with diverse backgrounds and special needs. (See A.2.a.)

F.3. Students and Supervisees

a. Limitations. Counselors, through ongoing evaluation and appraisal, are aware of the academic and personal limitations of students and supervisees that might impede performance. Counselors assist students and supervisees in securing remedial assistance when needed, and dismiss from the training program supervisees who are unable to provide competent service due to academic or personal limitations. Counselors seek professional consultation and document their decision to dismiss or refer students or supervisees for assistance. Counselors ensure that students and supervisees have recourse to address decisions made to require them to seek assistance or to dismiss them.

b. Self-Growth Experiences. Counselors use professional judgment when designing training experiences conducted by the counselors themselves that require student and supervisee self-growth or self-disclosure. Safeguards are provided so that students and supervisees are aware of the ramifications their self-disclosure may have on counselors whose primary role as teacher, trainer, or supervisor requires acting on ethical obligations to the profession. Evaluative components of experiential training experiences explicitly delineate predetermined academic standards that are separate and do not depend on the student's level of self-disclosure. (See A.6.)

c. Counseling for Students and Supervisees. If students or supervisees request counseling, supervisors or counselor educators provide them with acceptable referrals. Supervisors or counselor educators do not serve as counselor to students or supervisees over whom they hold administrative, teaching, or evaluative roles unless this is a brief role associated with a training experience. (See A.6.b.)

d. Clients of Students and Supervisees. Counselors make every effort to ensure that the clients at field placements are aware of the services rendered and the qualifications of the students and supervisees rendering those services. Clients receive professional disclosure information and are informed of the limits of confidentiality. Client permission is obtained in order for the students and supervisees to use any information concerning the counseling relationship in the training process. (See B.1.e.)

e. Standards for Students and Supervisees. Students and supervisees preparing to become counselors adhere to the Code of Ethics and the Standards of Practice. Students and supervisees have the same obligations to clients as those required of counselors. (See H.1.)

SECTION G: RESEARCH AND PUBLICATION

G.1. Research Responsibilities

a. Use of Human Subjects. Counselors plan, design, conduct, and report research in a manner consistent with pertinent ethical principles, federal and state laws, host institutional regulations, and scientific standards governing research with human subjects. Counselors design and conduct research that reflects cultural sensitivity appropriateness.

b. Deviation From Standard Practices. Counselors seek consultation and observe stringent safeguards to protect the rights of research participants when a research problem suggests a deviation from standard acceptable practices. (See B.6.)

c. Precautions to Avoid Injury. Counselors who conduct research with human subjects are responsible for the subjects' welfare throughout the experiment and take reasonable precautions to avoid causing injurious psychological, physical, or social effects to their subjects.

d. Principal Researcher Responsibility. The ultimate responsibility for ethical research practice lies with the principal researcher. All others involved in the research activities share ethical obligations and full responsibility for their own actions.

e. Minimal Interference. Counselors take reasonable precautions to avoid causing disruptions in subjects' lives due to participation in research.

f. Diversity. Counselors are sensitive to diversity and research issues with special populations. They seek consultation when appropriate. (See A.2.a. and B.6.)

G.2. Informed Consent

a. Topics Disclosed. In obtaining informed consent for research, counselors use language that is understandable to research participants and that (1) accurately explains the purpose and procedures to be followed; (2) identifies any procedures that are experimental or relatively untried; (3) describes the attendant discomforts and risks; (4) describes the benefits or changes in individuals or organizations that might be reasonably expected; (5) discloses appropriate alternative procedures that would be advantageous for subjects; (6) offers to answer any inquiries concerning the procedures; (7) describes any limitations on confidentiality; and (8) instructs that subjects are free to withdraw their consent and to discontinue participation in the project at any time. (See B.1.f.)

b.   Deception. Counselors do not conduct research involving deception unless alternative procedures are not feasible and the prospective value of the research justifies the deception. When the methodological requirements of a study necessitate concealment or deception, the investigator is required to explain clearly the reasons for this action as soon as possible.

c.   Voluntary Participation. Participation in research is typically voluntary and without any penalty for refusal to participate. Involuntary participation is appropriate only when it can be demonstrated that participation will have no harmful effects on subjects and is essential to the investigation.

d.   Confidentiality of Information. Information obtained about research participants during the course of an investigation is confidential. When the possibility exists that others may obtain access to such information, ethical research practice requires that the possibility, together with the plans for protecting confidentiality, be explained to participants as a part of the procedure for obtaining informed consent. (See B.1.e.)

e.   Persons Incapable of Giving Informed Consent. When a person is incapable of giving informed consent, counselors provide an appropriate explanation, obtain agreement for participation, and obtain appropriate consent from a legally authorized person.

f.   Commitments to Participants. Counselors take reasonable measures to honor all commitments to research participants.

g.   Explanations After Data Collection. After data are collected, counselors provide participants with full clarification of the nature of the study to remove any misconceptions. Where scientific or human values justify delaying or withholding information, counselors take reasonable measures to avoid causing harm.

h.   Agreements to Cooperate. Counselors who agree to cooperate with another individual in research or publication incur an obligation to cooperate as promised in terms of punctuality of performance and with regard to the completeness and accuracy of the information required.

i.   Informed Consent for Sponsors. In the pursuit of research, counselors give sponsors, institutions, and publication channels the same respect and opportunity for giving informed consent that they accord to individual research participants. Counselors are aware of their obligation to future research workers and ensure that host institutions are given feedback information and proper acknowledgment.

G.3. Reporting Results

a. Information Affecting Outcome. When reporting research results, counselors explicitly mention all variables and conditions known to the investigator that may have affected the outcome of a study or the interpretation of data.

b. Accurate Results. Counselors plan, conduct, and report research accurately and in a manner that minimizes the possibility that results will be misleading. They provide thorough discussions of the limitations of their data and alternative hypotheses. Counselors do not engage in fraudulent research, distort data, misrepresent data, or deliberately bias their results.

c. Obligation to Report Unfavorable Results. Counselors communicate to other counselors the results of any research judged to be of professional value. Results that reflect unfavorably on institutions, programs, services, prevailing opinions, or vested interests are not withheld.

d. Identity of Subjects. Counselors who supply data, aid in the research of another person, report research results, or make original data available take due care to disguise the identity of respective subjects in the absence of specific authorization from the subjects to do otherwise. (See B.1.g. and B.5.a.)

e. Replication Studies. Counselors are obligated to make available sufficient original research data to qualified professionals who may wish to replicate the study.

G.4. Publication

a. Recognition of Others. When conducting and reporting research, counselors are familiar with and give recognition to previous work on the topic, observe copyright laws, and give full credit to those to whom credit is due. (See F.1.d. and G.4.c.)

b. Contributors. Counselors give credit through joint authorship, acknowledgment, footnote statements, or other appropriate means to those who have contributed significantly to research or concept development in accordance with such contributions. The principal contributor is listed first and minor technical or professional contributions are acknowledged in notes or introductory statements.

c. Student Research. For an article that is substantially based on a student's dissertation or thesis, the student is listed as the principal author. (See F.1.d. and G.4.a.)

d. Duplicate Submission. Counselors submit manuscripts for consideration to only one journal at a time. Manuscripts that are

published in whole or in substantial part in another journal or
published work are not submitted for publication without acknowledgment and permission from the previous publication.

  e. Professional Review. Counselors who review material sub-
     mitted for publication, research, or other scholarly purposes
     respect the confidentiality and proprietary rights of those who
     submitted it.

SECTION H: RESOLVING ETHICAL ISSUES

H.1. Knowledge of Standards

Counselors are familiar with the Code of Ethics and the Standards of
Practice and other applicable ethics codes from other professional organizations of which they are member, or from certification and licensure
bodies. Lack of knowledge or misunderstanding of an ethical responsibility is not a defense against a charge of unethical conduct. (See F.3.e.)

H.2. Suspected Violations

  a. Ethical Behavior Expected. Counselors expect professional as-
     sociates to adhere to the Code of Ethics. When counselors pos-
     sess reasonable cause that raises doubts as to whether a coun-
     selor is acting in an ethical manner, they take appropriate action.
     (See H.2.d. and H.2.e.)
  b. Consultation. When uncertain as to whether a particular situa-
     tion or course of action may be in violation of the Code of
     Ethics, counselors consult with other counselors who are
     knowledgeable about ethics, with colleagues, or with appropri-
     ate authorities.
  c. Organization Conflicts. If the demands of an organization with
     which counselors are affiliated pose a conflict with the Code of
     Ethics, counselors specify the nature of such conflicts and ex-
     press to their supervisors or other responsible officials their com-
     mitment to the Code of Ethics. When possible, counselors work
     toward change within the organization to allow full adherence
     to the Code of Ethics.
  d. Informal Resolution. When counselors have reasonable cause
     to believe that another counselor is violating an ethical standard,
     they attempt to first resolve the issue informally with the other
     counselor if feasible, providing that such action does not violate
     confidentiality rights that may be involved.
  e. Reporting Suspected Violations. When an informal resolution is
     not appropriate or feasible, counselors, upon reasonable cause,

take action such as reporting the suspected ethical violation to state or national ethics committees, unless this action conflicts with confidentiality rights that cannot be resolved.

f. Unwarranted Complaints. Counselors do not initiate, participate in, or encourage the filing of ethics complaints that are unwarranted or intend to harm a counselor rather than to protect clients or the public.

H.3. Cooperation With Ethics Committees

Counselors assist in the process of enforcing the Code of Ethics. Counselors cooperate with investigations, proceedings, and requirements of the ACA Ethics Committee or ethics committees of other duly constituted associations or boards having jurisdiction over those charged with a violation. Counselors are familiar with the ACA Policies and Procedures and use it as a reference in assisting the enforcement of the Code of Ethics.

STANDARDS OF PRACTICE

All members of the American Counseling Association (ACA) are required to adhere to the Standards of Practice and the Code of Ethics. The Standards of Practice represent minimal behavioral statements of the Code of Ethics. Members should refer to the applicable section of the Code of Ethics for further interpretation and amplification of the applicable Standard of Practice.

Section A: The Counseling Relationship

Standard of Practice One (SP-1): Nondiscrimination. Counselors respect diversity and must not discriminate against clients because of age, color, culture, disability, ethnic group, gender, race, religion, sexual orientation, marital status, or socioeconomic status. (See A.2.a.)

Standard of Practice Two (SP-2): Disclosure to Clients. Counselors must adequately inform clients, preferably in writing, regarding the counseling process and counseling relationship at or before the time it begins and throughout the relationship. (See A.3.a.)

Standard of Practice Three (SP-3): Dual Relationships. Counselors must make every effort to avoid dual relationships with clients that could impair their professional judgment or increase the risk of harm to clients. When a dual relationship cannot be avoided, counselors must take appropriate steps to ensure that judgment is not impaired and that no exploitation occurs. (See A.6.a. and A.6.b.)

Standard of Practice Four (SP-4): Sexual Intimacies With Clients. Counselors must not engage in any type of sexual intimacies with current clients and must not engage in sexual intimacies with former clients within a minimum of 2 years after terminating the counseling relationship. Counselors who engage in such relationship after 2 years following termination have the responsibility to examine and document thoroughly that such relations did not have an exploitative nature.

Standard of Practice Five (SP-5): Protecting Clients During Group Work. Counselors must take steps to protect clients from physical or psychological trauma resulting from interactions during group work. (See A.9.b.)

Standard of Practice Six (SP-6): Advance Understanding of Fees. Counselors must explain to clients, prior to their entering the counseling relationship, financial arrangements related to professional services. (See A.10. a.-d. and A.11.c.)

Standard of Practice Seven (SP-7): Termination. Counselors must assist in making appropriate arrangements for the continuation of treatment of clients, when necessary, following termination of counseling relationships. (See A.11.a.)

Standard of Practice Eight (SP-8): Inability to Assist Clients. Counselors must avoid entering or immediately terminate a counseling relationship if it is determined that they are unable to be of professional assistance to a client. The counselor may assist in making an appropriate referral for the client. (See A.11.b.)

Section B: Confidentiality

Standard of Practice Nine (SP-9): Confidentiality Requirement. Counselors must keep information related to counseling services confidential unless disclosure is in the best interest of clients, is required for the welfare of others, or is required by law. When disclosure is required, only information that is essential is revealed and the client is informed of such disclosure. (See B.1. a.+ f.)

Standard of Practice Ten (SP-10): Confidentiality Requirements for Subordinates. Counselors must take measures to ensure that privacy and confidentiality of clients are maintained by subordinates. (See B.1.h.)

Standard of Practice Eleven (SP-11): Confidentiality in Group Work. Counselors must clearly communicate to group members that confidentiality cannot be guaranteed in group work. (See B.2.a.)

Standard of Practice Twelve (SP-12): Confidentiality in Family Counseling. Counselors must not disclose information about one family member in counseling to another family member without prior consent. (See B.2.b.)

Standard of Practice Thirteen (SP-13): Confidentiality of Records. Counselors must maintain appropriate confidentiality in creating, storing, accessing, transferring, and disposing of counseling records. (See B.4.b.)

Standard of Practice Fourteen (SP-14): Permission to Record or Observe. Counselors must obtain prior consent from clients in order to record electronically or observe sessions. (See B.4.c.)

Standard of Practice Fifteen (SP-15): Disclosure or Transfer of Records. Counselors must obtain client consent to disclose or transfer records to third parties, unless exceptions listed in SP-9 exist. (See B.4.e.)

Standard of Practice Sixteen (SP-16): Data Disguise Required. Counselors must disguise the identity of the client when using data for training, research, or publication. (See B.5.a.)

Section C: Professional Responsibility

Standard of Practice Seventeen (SP-17): Boundaries of Competence. Counselors must practice only within the boundaries of their competence. (See C.2.a.)

Standard of Practice Eighteen (SP-18): Continuing Education. Counselors must engage in continuing education to maintain their professional competence. (See C.2.f.)

Standard of Practice Nineteen (SP-19): Impairment of Professionals. Counselors must refrain from offering professional services when their personal problems or conflicts may cause harm to a client or others. (See C.2.g.)

Standard of Practice Twenty (SP-20): Accurate Advertising. Counselors must accurately represent their credentials and services when advertising. (See C.3.a.)

Standard of Practice Twenty-One (SP-21): Recruiting Through Employment. Counselors must not use their place of employment or institutional affiliation to recruit clients for their private practices. (See C.3.d.)

Standard of Practice Twenty-Two (SP-22): Credentials Claimed. Counselors must claim or imply only professional credentials possessed and must correct any known misrepresentations of their credentials by others. (See C.4.a.)

Standard of Practice Twenty-Three (SP-23): Sexual Harassment. Counselors must not engage in sexual harassment. (See C.5.b.)

Standard of Practice Twenty-Four (SP-24): Unjustified Gains. Counselors must not use their professional positions to seek or receive unjustified personal gains, sexual favors, unfair advantage, or unearned goods or services. (See C.5.e.)

Standard of Practice Twenty-Five (SP-25): Clients Served by Others. With the consent of the client, counselors must inform other mental health professionals serving the same client that a counseling relationship between the counselor and client exists. (See C.6.c.)

Standard of Practice Twenty-Six (SP-26): Negative Employment Conditions. Counselors must alert their employers to institutional policy or conditions that may be potentially disruptive or damaging to the counselor's professional responsibilities, or that may limit their effectiveness or deny clients' rights. (See D.1.c.)

Standard of Practice Twenty-Seven (SP-27): Personnel Selection and Assignment. Counselors must select competent staff and must assign responsibilities compatible with staff skills and experiences. (See D.1.h.)

Standard of Practice Twenty-Eight (SP-28): Exploitative Relationships With Subordinates. Counselors must not engage in exploitative relationships with individuals over whom they have supervisory, evaluative, or instructional control or authority. (See D.1.k.)

Section D: Relationship With Other Professionals

Standard of Practice Twenty-Nine (SP-29): Accepting Fees From Agency Clients. Counselors must not accept fees or other remuneration for consultation with persons entitled to such services through the counselor's employing agency or institution. (See D.3.a.)

Standard of Practice Thirty (SP-30): Referral Fees. Counselors must not accept referral fees. (See D.3.b.)

Section E: Evaluation, Assessment and Interpretation

Standard of Practice Thirty-One (SP-31): Limits of Competence. Counselors must perform only testing and assessment services for which they are competent. Counselors must not allow the use of psychological assessment techniques by unqualified persons under their supervision. (See E.2.a.)

Standard of Practice Thirty-Two (SP-32): Appropriate Use of Assessment Instruments. Counselors must use assessment instruments in the manner for which they were intended. (See E.2.b.)

Standard of Practice Thirty-Three (SP-33): Assessment Explanations to Clients. Counselors must provide explanations to clients prior to assessment about the nature and purposes of assessment and the specific uses of results. (See E.3.a.)

Standard of Practice Thirty-Four (SP-34): Recipients of Test Results. Counselors must ensure that accurate and appropriate interpretations accompany any release of testing and assessment information. (See E.3.b.)

Standard of Practice Thirty-Five (SP-35): Obsolete Tests and Outdated Test Results. Counselors must not base their assessment or intervention decisions or recommendations on data or test results that are obsolete or outdated for the current purpose. (See E.11.)

Section F: Teaching, Training, and Supervision

Standard of Practice Thirty-Six (SP-36): Sexual Relationships With Students or Supervisees. Counselors must not engage in sexual relationships with their students and supervisees. (See F.1.c.)

Standard of Practice Thirty-Seven (SP-37): Credit for Contributions to Research. Counselors must give credit to students or supervisees for their contributions to research and scholarly projects. (See F.1.d.)

Standard of Practice Thirty-Eight (SP-38): Supervision Preparation. Counselors who offer clinical supervision services must be trained and prepared in supervision methods and techniques. (See F.1.f.)

Standard of Practice Thirty-Nine (SP-39): Evaluation Information. Counselors must clearly state to students and supervisees in advance of training the levels of competency expected, appraisal methods, and timing of evaluations. Counselors must provide students and supervisees with periodic performance appraisal and evaluation feedback throughout the training program. (See F.2.c.)

Standard of Practice Forty (SP-40): Peer Relationships in Training. Counselors must make every effort to ensure that the rights of peers are not violated when students and supervisees are assigned to lead counseling groups or provide clinical supervision. (See F.2.e.)

Standard of Practice Forty-One (SP-41): Limitations of Students and Supervisees. Counselors must assist students and supervisees in securing remedial assistance, when needed, and must dismiss from the training program students and supervisees who are unable to provide competent service due to academic or personal limitations. (See F.3.a.)

Standard of Practice Forty-Two (SP-42): Self-Growth Experiences. Counselors who conduct experiences for students or supervisees that include self-growth or self-disclosure must inform participants of counselors' ethical obligations to the profession and must not grade participants based on their nonacademic performance. (See F.3.b.)

Standard of Practice Forty-Three (SP-43): Standards for Students and Supervisees. Students and supervisees preparing to become counselors must adhere to the Code of Ethics and the Standards of Practice of counselors. (See F.3.e.)

Section G: Research and Publication

Standard of Practice Forty-Four (SP-44): Precautions to Avoid Injury in Research. Counselors must avoid causing physical, social, or psychological harm or injury to subjects in research. (See G.1.c.)

Standard of Practice Forty-Five (SP-45): Confidentiality of Research Information. Counselors must keep confidential information obtained about research participants. (See G.2.d.)

Standard of Practice Forty-Six (SP-46): Information Affecting Research Outcome. Counselors must report all variables and conditions known to the investigator that may have affected research data or outcomes. (See G.3.a.)

Standard of Practice Forty-Seven (SP-47): Accurate Research Results. Counselors must not distort or misrepresent research data, nor fabricate or intentionally bias research results. (See G.3.b.)

Standard of Practice Forty-Eight (SP-48): Publication Contributors. Counselors must give appropriate credit to those who have contributed to research. (See G.4.a. and G.4.b.)

Section H: Resolving Ethical Issues

Standard of Practice Forty-Nine (SP-49): Ethical Behavior Expected. Counselors must take appropriate action when they possess reasonable cause that raises doubts as to whether counselors or other mental health professionals are acting in an ethical manner. (See H.2.a.)

Standard of Practice Fifty (SP-50): Unwarranted Complaints. Counselors must not initiate, participate in, or encourage the filing of ethics complaints that are unwarranted or intended to harm a mental health professional rather than to protect clients or the public. (See H.2.f.)

Standard of Practice Fifty-One (SP-51): Cooperation With Ethics Committees. Counselors must cooperate with investigations, proceedings, and requirements of the ACA Ethics Committee or ethics committees of other duly constituted associations or boards having jurisdiction over those charged with a violation. (See H.3.)

References

The following documents are available to counselors as resources to guide them in their practices. These resources are not a part of the Code of Ethics and the Standards of Practice.

American Association for Counseling and Development/Association for Measurement and Evaluation in Counseling and Development. (1989). The responsibilities of users of standardized tests (rev.). Washington, DC: Author.

American Counseling Association. (1988). Ethical standards. Alexandria, VA: Author.

American Psychological Association. (1985). Standards for educational and psychological testing (rev.). Washington, DC: Author.

American Rehabilitation Counseling Association, Commission on Rehabilitation Counselor Certification, and National Rehabilitation Counseling Association. (1995). Code of professional ethics for rehabilitation counselors. Chicago, IL: Author.

American School Counselor Association. (1992). Ethical standards for school counselors. Alexandria, VA: Author.

Joint Committee on Testing Practices. (1988). Code of fair testing practices in education. Washington, DC: Author.

National Board for Certified Counselors. (1989). National Board for Certified Counselors code of ethics. Alexandria, VA: Author.

Prediger, D. J. (Ed.). (1993, March). Multicultural assessment standards. Alexandria, VA: Association for Assessment in Counseling.

Appendix C

THE PRINCIPLES OF MEDICAL ETHICS
WITH ANNOTATIONS ESPECIALLY
APPLICABLE TO PSYCHIATRY
American Psychiatric Association*

In 1973, the American Psychiatric Association (APA) published the first edition of *The Principles of Medical Ethics With Annotations Especially Applicable to Psychiatry.* Subsequently, revisions were published as the APA Board of Trustees and the APA Assembly approved additional annotations. In July of 1980, the American Medical Association (AMA) approved a new version of the *Principles of Medical Ethics* (the first revision since 1957), and the APA Ethics Committee[1] incorporated many of its annotations into the new *Principles,* which resulted in the 1981 edition and subsequent revisions.

FOREWORD

ALL PHYSICIANS should practice in accordance with the medical code of ethics set forth in the *Principles of Medical Ethics* of the American Medical Association. An up-to-date expression and elaboration of

---

*From *The Principles of Medical Ethics With Annotations Especially Applicable to Psychiatry.* Copyright © 2001 by the American Psychiatric Publishing, Inc. (www.appi.org). Reprinted with permission.

[1]The committee included Herbert Klemmer, M.D., Chairperson, Miltiades Zaphiropoulos, M.D., Ewald Busse, M.D., John R. Saunders, M.D., and Robert McDevitt, M.D. J. Brand Brickman, M.D., William P. Camp, M.D., and Robert A. Moore, M.D., served as consultants to the APA Ethics Committee.

these statements is found in the Opinions and Reports of the Council on Ethical and Judicial Affairs of the American Medical Association.[2] Psychiatrists are strongly advised to be familiar with these documents.[3]

However, these general guidelines have sometimes been difficult to interpret for psychiatry, so further annotations to the basic principles are offered in this document. While psychiatrists have the same goals as all physicians, there are special ethical problems in psychiatric practice that differ in coloring and degree from ethical problems in other branches of medical practice, even though the basic principles are the same. The annotations are not designed as absolutes and will be revised from time to time so as to be applicable to current practices and problems.

Following are the AMA *Principles of Medical Ethics,* printed in their entirety, and then each principle printed separately along with an annotation especially applicable to psychiatry.

PRINCIPLES OF MEDICAL ETHICS
American Medical Association

PREAMBLE

The medical profession has long subscribed to a body of ethical statements developed primarily for the benefit of the patient. As a member of this profession, a physician must recognize responsibility not only to patients, but also to society, to other health professionals, and to self. The following Principles adopted by the American Medical Association are not laws, but standards of conduct which define the essentials of honorable behavior for the physician.

Section 1

A physician shall be dedicated to providing competent medical service with compassion and respect for human dignity.

---

[2] *Current Opinions With Annotations of the Council on Ethical and Judicial Affiars,* Chicago, American Medical Association, 2000-2001.

[3] Chapter 8, Section 1 of the Bylaws of the American Psychiatric Association states, "All members of the Association shall be bound by the ethical code of the medical profession, specifically defined in the *Principles of Medical Ethics* of the American Medical Association and in the Association's *Principles of Medical Ethics With Annotations Especially Applicable to Psychiatry.*" In interpreting the Bylaws, it is the opinion of the APA Board of Trustees that inactive status in no way removes a physician member from responsibility to abide by the *Principles of Medical Ethics.*

Section 2

A physician shall deal honestly with patients and colleagues, and strive to expose those physicians deficient in character or competence, or who engage in fraud or deception.

Section 3

A physician shall respect the law and also recognize a responsibility to seek changes in those requirements which are contrary to the best interests of the patient.

Section 4

A physician shall respect the rights of patients, of colleagues, and of other health professionals, and shall safeguard patient confidences within the constraints of the law.

Section 5

A physician shall continue to study, apply, and advance scientific knowledge, make relevant information available to patients, colleagues, and the public, obtain consultation, and use the talents of other health professionals when indicated.

Section 6

A physician shall, in the provision of appropriate patient care, except in emergencies, be free to choose whom to serve, with whom to associate, and the environment in which to provide medical services.

Section 7

A physician shall recognize a responsibility to participate in activities contributing to an improved community.

PRINCIPLES WITH ANNOTATIONS

Following are each of the AMA *Principles of Medical Ethics* printed separately along with annotations especially applicable to psychiatry.

PREAMBLE

The medical profession has long subscribed to a body of ethical statements developed primarily for the benefit of the patient. As a member of this profession, a physician must recognize responsibility not only to patients, but also to society, to other health professionals, and to self. The following Principles adopted by the American Medical Association are not laws, but standards of conduct which define the essentials of honorable behavior for the physician.

Section 1

A physician shall be dedicated to providing competent medical service with compassion and respect for human dignity.

1. A psychiatrist shall not gratify his/her own needs by exploiting the patient. The psychiatrist shall be ever vigilant about the impact that his/her conduct has upon the boundaries of the doctor-patient relationship, and thus upon the well-being of the patient. These requirements become particularly important because of the essentially private, highly personal, and sometimes intensely emotional nature of the relationship established with the psychiatrist.

2. A psychiatrist should not be a party to any type of policy that excludes, segregates, or demeans the dignity of any patient because of ethnic origin, race, sex, creed, age, socioeconomic status, or sexual orientation.

3. In accord with the requirements of law and accepted medical practice, it is ethical for a physician to submit his/her work to peer review and to the ultimate authority of the medical staff executive body and the hospital administration and its governing body. In case of dispute, the ethical psychiatrist has the following steps available:

   A. Seek appeal from the medical staff decision to a joint conference committee, including members of the medical staff executive committee and the executive committee of the governing board. At this appeal, the ethical psychiatrist could request that outside opinions be considered.
   B. Appeal to the governing body itself.
   C. Appeal to state agencies regulating licensure of hospitals if, in the particular state, they concern themselves with matters of professional competency and quality of care.
   D. Attempt to educate colleagues through development of research projects and data and presentations at professional meetings and in professional journals.
   E. Seek redress in local courts, perhaps through an enjoining injunction against the governing body.

F. Public education as carried out by an ethical psychiatrist would not utilize appeals based solely upon emotion, but would be presented in a professional way and without any potential exploitation of patients through testimonials.

4. A psychiatrist should not be a participant in a legally authorized execution.

Section 2

A physician shall deal honestly with patients and colleagues, and strive to expose those physicians deficient in character or competence, or who engage in fraud or deception.

1. The requirement that the physician conduct himself/herself with propriety in his/her profession and in all the actions of his/her life is especially important in the case of the psychiatrist because the patient tends to model his/her behavior after that of his/her psychiatrist by identification. Further, the necessary intensity of the treatment relationship may tend to activate sexual and other needs and fantasies on the part of both patient and psychiatrist, while weakening the objectivity necessary for control. Additionally, the inherent inequality in the doctor-patient relationship may lead to exploitation of the patient. Sexual activity with a current or former patient is unethical.

2. The psychiatrist should diligently guard against exploiting information furnished by the patient and should not use the unique position of power afforded him/her by the psychotherapeutic situation to influence the patient in any way not directly relevant to the treatment goals.

3. A psychiatrist who regularly practices outside his/her area of professional competence should be considered unethical. Determination of professional competence should be made by peer review boards or other appropriate bodies.

4. Special consideration should be given to those psychiatrists who, because of mental illness, jeopardize the welfare of their patients and their own reputations and practices. It is ethical, even encouraged, for another psychiatrist to intercede in such situations.

5. Psychiatric services, like all medical services, are dispensed in the context of a contractual arrangement between the patient and the physician. The provisions of the contractual arrangement, which are binding on the physician as well as on the patient, should be explicitly established.

6. It is ethical for the psychiatrist to make a charge for a missed appointment when this falls within the terms of the specific contractual agreement with the patient. Charging for a missed appointment or for one not canceled 24 hours in advance need not, in itself, be considered unethical if a patient is fully advised that the physician will make such a charge. The practice, however, should be resorted to infrequently and always with the utmost consideration for the patient and his/her circumstances.

7. An arrangement in which a psychiatrist provides supervision or administration to other physicians or nonmedical persons for a percentage of their fees or gross income is not acceptable; this would constitute fee splitting. In a team of practitioners, or a multidisciplinary team, it is ethical for the psychiatrist to receive income for administration, research, education, or consultation. This should be based on a mutually agreed-upon and set fee or salary, open to renegotiation when a change in the time demand occurs. (See also Section 5, Annotations 2, 3, and 4.)

Section 3

A physician shall respect the law and also recognize a responsibility to seek changes in those requirements which are contrary to the best interests of the patient.

1. It would seem self-evident that a psychiatrist who is a lawbreaker might be ethically unsuited to practice his/her profession. When such illegal activities bear directly upon his/her practice, this would obviously be the case. However, in other instances, illegal activities such as those concerning the right to protest social injustices might not bear on either the image of the psychiatrist or the ability of the specific psychiatrist to treat his/her patient ethically and well. While no committee or board could offer prior assurance that any illegal activity would not be considered unethical, it is conceivable that an individual could violate a law without being guilty of professionally unethical behavior. Physicians lose no right of citizenship on entry into the profession of medicine.

2. Where not specifically prohibited by local laws governing medical practice, the practice of acupuncture by a psychiatrist is not unethical per se. The psychiatrist should have professional competence in the use of acupuncture. Or, if he/she is supervising the use of acupuncture by nonmedical individuals, he/she should

provide proper medical supervision. (See also Section 5, Annotations 3 and 4.)

Section 4

A physician shall respect the rights of patients, of colleagues, and of other health professionals, and shall safeguard patient confidences within the constraints of the law.

1. Psychiatric records, including even the identification of a person as a patient, must be protected with extreme care. Confidentiality is essential to psychiatric treatment. This is based in part on the special nature of psychiatric therapy as well as on the traditional ethical relationship between physician and patient. Growing concern regarding the civil rights of patients and the possible adverse effects of computerization, duplication equipment, and data banks makes the dissemination of confidential information an increasing hazard. Because of the sensitive and private nature of the information with which the psychiatrist deals, he/she must be circumspect in the information that he/she chooses to disclose to others about a patient. The welfare of the patient must be a continuing consideration.

2. A psychiatrist may release confidential information only with the authorization of the patient or under proper legal compulsion. The continuing duty of the psychiatrist to protect the patient includes fully apprising him/her of the connotations of waiving the privilege of privacy. This may become an issue when the patient is being investigated by a government agency, is applying for a position, or is involved in legal action. The same principles apply to the release of information concerning treatment to medical departments of government agencies, business organizations, labor unions, and insurance companies. Information gained in confidence about patients seen in student health services should not be released without the students' explicit permission.

3. Clinical and other materials used in teaching and writing must be adequately disguised in order to preserve the anonymity of the individuals involved.

4. The ethical responsibility of maintaining confidentiality holds equally for the consultations in which the patient may not have been present and in which the consultee was not a physician. In such instances, the physician consultant should alert the consultee to his/her duty of confidentiality.

5. Ethically, the psychiatrist may disclose only that information which is relevant to a given situation. He/she should avoid offering speculation as fact. Sensitive information such as an individual's sexual orientation or fantasy material is usually unnecessary.

6. Psychiatrists are often asked to examine individuals for security purposes, to determine suitability for various jobs, and to determine legal competence. The psychiatrist must fully describe the nature and purpose and lack of confidentiality of the examination to the examinee at the beginning of the examination.

7. Careful judgment must be exercised by the psychiatrist in order to include, when appropriate, the parents or guardian in the treatment of a minor. At the same time, the psychiatrist must assure the minor proper confidentiality.

8. Psychiatrists at times may find it necessary, in order to protect the patient or the community from imminent danger, to reveal confidential information disclosed by the patient.

9. When the psychiatrist is ordered by the court to reveal the confidences entrusted to him/her by patients, he/she may comply or he/she may ethically hold the right to dissent within the framework of the law. When the psychiatrist is in doubt, the right of the patient to confidentiality and, by extension, to unimpaired treatment should be given priority. The psychiatrist should reserve the right to raise the question of adequate need for disclosure. In the event that the necessity for legal disclosure is demonstrated by the court, the psychiatrist may request the right to disclosure of only that information which is relevant to the legal question at hand.

10. With regard for the person's dignity and privacy and with truly informed consent, it is ethical to present a patient to a scientific gathering if the confidentiality of the presentation is understood and accepted by the audience.

11. It is ethical to present a patient or former patient to a public gathering or to the news media only if the patient is fully informed of enduring loss of confidentiality, is competent, and consents in writing without coercion.

12. When involved in funded research, the ethical psychiatrist will advise human subjects of the funding source, retain his/her freedom to reveal data and results, and follow all appropriate and current guidelines relative to human subject protection.

13. Ethical considerations in medical practice preclude the psychiatric evaluation of any person charged with criminal acts prior to access to, or availability of, legal counsel. The only exception is

the rendering of care to the person for the sole purpose of medical treatment.

14. Sexual involvement between a faculty member or supervisor and a trainee or student, in those situations in which an abuse of power can occur, often takes advantage of inequalities in the working relationship and may be unethical because

   A. Any treatment of a patient being supervised may be deleteriously affected.
   B. It may damage the trust relationship between teacher and student.
   C. Teachers are important professional role models for their trainees and affect their trainees' future professional behavior.

Section 5

A physician shall continue to study, apply, and advance scientific knowledge, make relevant information available to patients, colleagues, and the public, obtain consultation, and use the talents of other health professionals when indicated.

1. Psychiatrists are responsible for their own continuing education and should be mindful of the fact that theirs must be a lifetime of learning.
2. In the practice of his/her specialty, the psychiatrist consults, associates, collaborates, or integrates his/her work with that of many professionals, including psychologists, psychometricians, social workers, alcoholism counselors, marriage counselors, public health nurses, and the like. Furthermore, the nature of modern psychiatric practice extends his/her contacts to such people as teachers, juvenile and adult probation officers, attorneys, welfare workers, agency volunteers, and neighborhood aides. In referring patients for treatment, counseling, or rehabilitation to any of these practitioners, the psychiatrist should ensure that the allied professional or paraprofessional with whom he/she is dealing is a recognized member of his/her own discipline and is competent to carry out the therapeutic task required. The psychiatrist should have the same attitude toward members of the medical profession to whom he/she refers patients. Whenever he/she has reason to doubt the training, skill, or ethical qualifications of the allied professional, the psychiatrist should not refer cases to him/her.

3. When the psychiatrist assumes a collaborative or supervisory role with another mental health worker, he/she must expend sufficient time to assure that proper care is given. It is contrary to the interests of the patient and to patient care if the psychiatrist allows himself/herself to be used as a figurehead.

4. In relationships between psychiatrists and practicing licensed psychologists, the physician should not delegate to the psychologist or, in fact, to any nonmedical person any matter requiring the exercise of professional medical judgment.

5. The psychiatrist should agree to the request of a patient for consultation or to such a request from the family of an incompetent or minor patient. The psychiatrist may suggest possible consultants, but the patient or family should be given free choice of the consultant. If the psychiatrist disapproves of the professional qualifications of the consultant or if there is a difference of opinion that the primary therapist cannot resolve, he/she may, after suitable notice, withdraw from the case. If this disagreement occurs within an institution or agency framework, the differences should be resolved by the mediation or arbitration of higher professional authority within the institution or agency.

Section 6

A physician shall, in the provision of appropriate patient care, except in emergencies, be free to choose whom to serve, with whom to associate, and the environment in which to provide medical services.

1. Physicians generally agree that the doctor-patient relationship is such a vital factor in effective treatment of the patient that preservation of optimal conditions for development of a sound working relationship between a doctor and his/her patient should take precedence over all other considerations. Professional courtesy may lead to poor psychiatric care for physicians and their families because of embarrassment over the lack of a complete give-and-take contract.

2. An ethical psychiatrist may refuse to provide psychiatric treatment to a person who, in the psychiatrist's opinion, cannot be diagnosed as having a mental illness amenable to psychiatric treatment.

Section 7

A physician shall recognize a responsibility to participate in activities contributing to an improved community.

1. Psychiatrists should foster the cooperation of those legitimately concerned with the medical, psychological, social, and legal aspects of mental health and illness. Psychiatrists are encouraged to serve society by advising and consulting with the executive, legislative, and judiciary branches of the government. A psychiatrist should clarify whether he/she speaks as an individual or as a representative of an organization. Furthermore, psychiatrists should avoid cloaking their public statements with the authority of the profession (e.g., "Psychiatrists know that . . .").

2. Psychiatrists may interpret and share with the public their expertise in the various psychosocial issues that may affect mental health and illness. Psychiatrists should always be mindful of their separate roles as dedicated citizens and as experts in psychological medicine.

3. On occasion psychiatrists are asked for an opinion about an individual who is in the light of public attention or who has disclosed information about himself/herself through public media. In such circumstances, a psychiatrist may share with the public his/her expertise about psychiatric issues in general. However, it is unethical for a psychiatrist to offer a professional opinion unless he/she has conducted an examination and has been granted proper authorization for such a statement.

4. The psychiatrist may permit his/her certification to be used for the involuntary treatment of any person only following his/her personal examination of that person. To do so, he/she must find that the person, because of mental illness, cannot form a judgment as to what is in his/her own best interests and that, without such treatment, substantial impairment is likely to occur to the person or others.

ADDENDUM TO
THE 2001 EDITION OF
THE PRINCIPLES OF MEDICAL ETHICS
WITH ANNOTATIONS ESPECIALLY
APPLICABLE TO PSYCHIATRY

Addendum 1

GUIDELINES FOR ETHICAL
PRACTICE IN ORGANIZED SETTINGS

At its meeting of September 13-14, 1997, the APA Ethics Committee voted to make the "Guidelines for Ethical Practice in Organized Settings," as approved by the Board and the Assembly, an addendum to *The Principles of Medical Ethics With Annotations Especially Applicable to Psychiatry,* to be preceded by introductory historical comments and cross-referenced to the appropriate annotations, as follows:

This addendum to *The Principles of Medical Ethics With Annotations Especially Applicable to Psychiatry* was approved by the Board of Trustees in March 1997 and by the Assembly of District Branches in May 1997. This addendum contains specific guidelines regarding ethical psychiatric practice in organized settings and is intended to clarify existing ethical standards contained in Sections 1-7.

ADDENDUM

Psychiatrists have a long and valued tradition of being essential participants in organizations that deliver health care. Such organizations can enhance medical effectiveness and protect the standards and values of the psychiatric profession by fostering competent, compassionate medical care in a setting in which informed consent and confidentiality are rigorously preserved, conditions essential for the successful treatment of mental illness. However, some organizations may place the psychiatrist in a position where the clinical needs of the patient, the demands of the community and larger society, and even the professional role of the psychiatrist are in conflict with the interests of the organization.

The psychiatrist must consider the consequences of such role conflicts with respect to patients in his or her care, and strive to resolve these conflicts in a manner that is likely to be of greatest benefit to the patient. Whether during treatment or a review process, a psychiatrist shall respect the autonomy, privacy, and dignity of the patient and his or her family.

These guidelines are intended to clarify existing standards. They are intended to promote the interests of the patient and should not be construed to interfere with the ability of a psychiatrist to practice in an organized setting. The principles and annotations noted in this communication conform to the statement in the preamble to the Principles of Medical Ethics. These are not laws but standards of conduct, which define the essentials of honorable behavior for the physician.

1. **Appropriateness of Treatment and Treatment Options**

    A. A psychiatrist shall not withhold information that the patient needs or reasonably could use to make informed treatment decisions, including options for treatment not provided by the psychiatrist. [Section 1, Annotation 1 (APA); Section 2, Annotation 4 (APA)]

    B. A psychiatrist's treatment plan shall be based upon clinical, scientific, or generally accepted standards of treatment. This applies to the treating and the reviewing psychiatrist. [Section 1, Annotation 1 (APA); Section 2 (APA); Section 4 (APA)]

    C. A psychiatrist shall strive to provide beneficial treatment that shall not be limited to minimum criteria of medical necessity. [Section 1, Annotation 1 (APA)]

2. **Financial Arrangements**

    When a psychiatrist is aware of financial incentives or penalties that limit the provision of appropriate treatment for that patient, the psychiatrist shall inform the patient and/or designated guardian. [Section 1, Annotation 1 (APA); Section 2 (APA)]

3. **Review Process**

    A psychiatrist shall not conduct reviews or participate in reviews in a manner likely to demean the dignity of the patient by asking for highly personal material not necessary for the conduct of the review. A reviewing psychiatrist shall strive as hard for a patient he or she reviews as for one he or she treats to prevent the disclosure of sensitive patient material to anyone other than for clear, clinical necessity. [Section 1, Annotations 1 and 2 (APA); Section 4, Annotations 1, 2, 4, and 5 (APA)]

Appendix D

ETHICAL PRINCIPLES OF PSYCHOLOGISTS AND CODE OF CONDUCT 2002
American Psychological Association*

INTRODUCTION AND APPLICABILITY

The American Psychological Association's (APA's) Ethical Principles of Psychologists and Code of Conduct (hereinafter referred to as the Ethics Code) consists of an Introduction, a Preamble, five General Prin-

*From "Ethical Principles of Psychologists and Code of Conduct" by the American Psychological Association. Copyright © 2002 by the American Psychological Association. Reprinted with permission.

This version of the APA Ethics Code was adopted by the American Psychological Association's Council of Representatives during its meeting, August 21, 2002, and is effective beginning June 1, 2003. Inquiries concerning the substance or interpretation of the APA Ethics Code should be addressed to the Director, Office of Ethics, American Psychological Association, 750 First Street, NE, Washington, DC 20002-4242. The Ethics Code and information regarding the Code can be found on the APA web site, http://www.apa.org/ethics. The standards in this Ethics Code will be used to adjudicate complaints brought concerning alleged conduct occurring on or after the effective date. Complaints regarding conduct occurring prior to the effective date will be adjudicated on the basis of the version of the Ethics Code that was in effect at the time the conduct occurred.

The APA has previously published its Ethics Code as follows:

American Psychological Association. (1953). *Ethical Standards of Psychologists*. Washington, DC: Author.

American Psychological Association. (1959). Ethical Standards of psychologists. *American Psychologist, 14*, 279-282.

American Psychological Association. (1963). Ethical Standards of psychologists. *American Psychologist, 18*, 56-60.

American Psychological Association. (1968). Ethical Standards of psychologists. *American Psychologist, 23*, 357-361.

American Psychological Association. (1977, March). Ethical Standards of psychologists. *APA Monitor*, pp. 22-23.

American Psychological Association. (1979). *Ethical Standards of Psychologists*. Washington, DC: Author.

American Psychological Association. (1981). Ethical principles of psychologists. *American Psychologist, 36*, 633-638.

American Psychological Association. (1990). Ethical principles of psychologists (Amended June 2, 1989). *American Psychologist, 45*, 390-395.

American Psychological Association. (1992). Ethical principles of psychologists and code of conduct. *American Psychologist, 47*, 1597-1611.

Request copies of the APA's *Ethical Principles of Psychologists and Code of Conduct* from the APA Order Department, 750 First Street, NE, Washington, DC 20002-4242, or phone (202) 336-5510.

ciples (A – E), and specific Ethical Standards. The Introduction discusses the intent, organization, procedural considerations, and scope of application of the Ethics Code. The Preamble and General Principles are aspirational goals to guide psychologists toward the highest ideals of psychology. Although the Preamble and General Principles are not themselves enforceable rules, they should be considered by psychologists in arriving at an ethical course of action. The Ethical Standards set forth enforceable rules for conduct as psychologists. Most of the Ethical Standards are written broadly, in order to apply to psychologists in varied roles, although the application of an Ethical Standard may vary depending on the context. The Ethical Standards are not exhaustive. The fact that a given conduct is not specifically addressed by an Ethical Standard does not mean that it is necessarily either ethical or unethical.

This Ethics Code applies only to psychologists' activities that are part of their scientific, educational, or professional roles as psychologists. Areas covered include but are not limited to the clinical, counseling, and school practice of psychology; research; teaching; supervision of trainees; public service; policy development; social intervention; development of assessment instruments; conducting assessments; educational counseling; organizational consulting; forensic activities; program design and evaluation; and administration. This Ethics Code applies to these activities across a variety of contexts, such as in person, postal, telephone, internet, and other electronic transmissions. These activities shall be distinguished from the purely private conduct of psychologists, which is not within the purview of the Ethics Code.

Membership in the APA commits members and student affiliates to comply with the standards of the APA Ethics Code and to the rules and procedures used to enforce them. Lack of awareness or misunderstanding of an Ethical Standard is not itself a defense to a charge of unethical conduct.

The procedures for filing, investigating, and resolving complaints of unethical conduct are described in the current Rules and Procedures of the APA Ethics Committee. APA may impose sanctions on its members for violations of the standards of the Ethics Code, including termination of APA membership, and may notify other bodies and individuals of its actions. Actions that violate the standards of the Ethics Code may also lead to the imposition of sanctions on psychologists or students whether or not they are APA members by bodies other than APA, including state psychological associations, other professional groups, psychology boards, other state or federal agencies, and payors for health services. In addition, APA may take action against a member after his or her conviction of a felony, expulsion or suspension from an affiliated state psychological association, or suspension or loss of licensure. When the sanction to be imposed by APA is less than expulsion, the 2001 Rules and Procedures do not guarantee an opportunity for an in-person hearing, but generally provide that complaints will be resolved only on the basis of a submitted record.

The Ethics Code is intended to provide guidance for psychologists and standards of professional conduct that can be applied by the APA and by other bodies that choose to adopt them. The Ethics Code is not intended to be a basis of civil liability. Whether a psychologist has violated the Ethics Code standards does not by itself determine whether the psychologist is legally liable in a court action, whether a contract is enforceable, or whether other legal consequences occur.

The modifiers used in some of the standards of this Ethics Code (e.g., *reasonably, appropriate, potentially*) are included in the standards when they would (1) allow professional judgment on the part of psychologists, (2) eliminate injustice or inequality that would occur without the modifier, (3) ensure applicability across the broad range of activities conducted by psychologists, or (4) guard against a set of rigid rules that might be quickly outdated. As used in this Ethics Code, the term *reasonable* means the prevailing professional judgment of psychologists engaged in similar activities in similar circumstances, given the knowledge the psychologist had or should have had at the time.

In the process of making decisions regarding their professional behavior, psychologists must consider this Ethics Code in addition to applicable laws and psychology board regulations. In applying the Ethics Code to their professional work, psychologists may consider other materials and guidelines that have been adopted or endorsed by scientific and professional psychological organizations and the dictates of their own conscience, as well as consult with others within the field. If this Ethics Code establishes a higher standard of conduct than is required by law, psychologists must meet the higher ethical standard. If psychologists' ethical responsibilities conflict with law, regulations, or other governing legal authority, psychologists make known their commitment to this Ethics Code and take steps to resolve the conflict in a responsible manner. If the conflict is unresolvable via such means, psychologists may adhere to the requirements of the law, regulations, or other governing authority in keeping with basic principles of human rights.

Preamble

Psychologists are committed to increasing scientific and professional knowledge of behavior and people's understanding of themselves and others and to the use of such knowledge to improve the condition of individuals, organizations, and society. Psychologists respect and protect civil and human rights and the central importance of freedom of inquiry and expression in research, teaching, and publication. They strive to help the public in developing informed judgments and choices concerning human behavior. In doing so, they perform many roles, such as researcher, educator, diagnostician, therapist, supervisor, consultant, administrator, social interventionist, and expert witness. This Ethics Code provides a common set of principles and standards upon which psychologists build their professional and scientific work.

This Ethics Code is intended to provide specific standards to cover most situations encountered by psychologists. It has as its goals the welfare and protection of the individuals and groups with whom psychologists work and the education of members, students, and the public regarding ethical standards of the discipline.

The development of a dynamic set of ethical standards for psychologists' work-related conduct requires a personal commitment and lifelong effort to act ethically; to encourage ethical behavior by students, supervisees, employees, and colleagues; and to consult with others concerning ethical problems.

GENERAL PRINCIPLES

This section consists of General Principles. General Principles, as opposed to Ethical Standards, are aspirational in nature. Their intent is to guide and inspire psychologists toward the very highest ethical ideals of the profession. General Principles, in contrast to Ethical Standards, do not represent obligations and should not form the basis for imposing sanctions. Relying upon General Principles for either of these reasons distorts both their meaning and purpose.

Principle A: Beneficence and Nonmaleficence

Psychologists strive to benefit those with whom they work and take care to do no harm. In their professional actions, psychologists seek to safeguard the welfare and rights of those with whom they interact professionally and other affected persons, and the welfare of animal subjects of research. When conflicts occur among psychologists' obligations or concerns, they attempt to resolve these conflicts in a responsible fashion that avoids or minimizes harm. Because psychologists' scientific and professional judgments and actions may affect the lives of others, they are alert to and guard against personal, financial, social, organizational, or political factors that might lead to misuse of their influence. Psychologists strive to be aware of the possible effect of their own physical and mental health on their ability to help those with whom they work.

Principle B: Fidelity and Responsibility

Psychologists establish relationships of trust with those with whom they work. They are aware of their professional and scientific responsibilities to society and to the specific communities in which they work. Psychologists uphold professional standards of conduct, clarify their professional roles and obligations, accept appropriate responsibility for their behavior, and seek to manage conflicts of interest that could lead to exploitation or harm. Psychologists consult with, refer to, or cooperate with other professionals and institutions to the extent needed to serve the best interests of those with whom they work. They are concerned about the ethical compliance of their colleagues' scientific and professional conduct. Psychologists strive to contribute a portion of their professional time for little or no compensation or personal advantage.

Principle C: Integrity

Psychologists seek to promote accuracy, honesty, and truthfulness in the science, teaching, and practice of psychology. In these activities psychologists do not steal, cheat, or engage in fraud, subterfuge, or intentional misrepresentation of fact. Psychologists strive to keep their promises and to avoid unwise or unclear commitments. In situations in which deception may be ethically justifiable to maximize benefits and minimize harm, psychologists have a serious obligation to consider the need for, the possible consequences of, and their responsibility to correct any resulting mistrust or other harmful effects that arise from the use of such techniques.

Principle D: Justice

Psychologists recognize that fairness and justice entitle all persons to access to and benefit from the contributions of psychology and to equal quality in the processes, procedures, and services being conducted by psychologists. Psychologists exercise reasonable judgment and take precautions to ensure that their potential biases, the boundaries of their competence, and the limitations of their expertise do not lead to or condone unjust practices.

Principle E: Respect for People's Rights and Dignity

Psychologists respect the dignity and worth of all people, and the rights of individuals to privacy, confidentiality, and self-determination. Psychologists are aware that special safeguards may be necessary to protect the rights and welfare of persons or communities whose vulnerabilities impair autonomous decision making. Psychologists are aware of and respect cultural, individual, and role differences, including those based on age, gender, gender identity, race, ethnicity, culture, national origin, religion, sexual orientation, disability, language, and socioeconomic status and consider these factors when working with members of such groups. Psychologists try to eliminate the effect on their work of biases based on those factors, and they do not knowingly participate in or condone activities of others based upon such prejudices.

ETHICAL STANDARDS

1. RESOLVING ETHICAL ISSUES

1.01   Misuse of Psychologists' Work

If psychologists learn of misuse or misrepresentation of their work, they take reasonable steps to correct or minimize the misuse or misrepresentation.

1.02   Conflicts Between Ethics and Law, Regulations, or Other Governing Legal Authority

If psychologists' ethical responsibilities conflict with law, regulations, or other governing legal authority, psychologists make known their commitment to the Ethics Code and take steps to resolve the conflict. If the conflict is unresolvable via such means, psychologists may adhere to the requirements of the law, regulations, or other governing legal authority.

1.03   Conflicts Between Ethics and Organizational Demands

If the demands of an organization with which psychologists are affiliated or for whom they are working conflict with this Ethics Code, psychologists clarify the nature of the conflict, make known their commitment to the Ethics Code, and to the extent feasible, resolve the conflict in a way that permits adherence to the Ethics Code.

1.04   Informal Resolution of Ethical Violations

When psychologists believe that there may have been an ethical violation by another psychologist, they attempt to resolve the issue by bringing it to the attention of that individual, if an informal resolution appears appropriate and the intervention does not violate any confidentiality rights that may be involved. (See also Standards 1.02, Conflicts Between Ethics and Law, Regulations, or Other Governing Legal Authority, and 1.03, Conflicts Between Ethics and Organizational Demands.)

1.05 Reporting Ethical Violations

If an apparent ethical violation has substantially harmed or is likely to substantially harm a person or organization and is not appropriate for informal resolution under Standard 1.04, Informal Resolution of Ethical Violations, or is not resolved properly in that fashion, psychologists take further action appropriate to the situation. Such action might include referral to state or national committees on professional ethics, to state licensing boards, or to the appropriate institutional authorities. This standard does not apply when an intervention would violate confidentiality rights or when psychologists have been retained to review the work of another psychologist whose professional conduct is in question. (See also Standard 1.02, Conflicts Between Ethics and Law, Regulations, or Other Governing Legal Authority.)

1.06 Cooperating With Ethics Committees

Psychologists cooperate in ethics investigations, proceedings, and resulting requirements of the APA or any affiliated state psychological association to which they belong. In doing so, they address any confidentiality issues. Failure to cooperate is itself an ethics violation. However, making a request for deferment of adjudication of an ethics complaint pending the outcome of litigation does not alone constitute noncooperation.

1.07 Improper Complaints

Psychologists do not file or encourage the filing of ethics complaints that are made with reckless disregard for or willful ignorance of facts that would disprove the allegation.

1.08 Unfair Discrimination Against Complainants and Respondents

Psychologists do not deny persons employment, advancement, admissions to academic or other programs, tenure, or promotion, based solely upon their having made or their being the subject of an ethics complaint. This does not preclude taking action based upon the outcome of such proceedings or considering other appropriate information.

2. COMPETENCE

2.01 Boundaries of Competence

(a) Psychologists provide services, teach, and conduct research with populations and in areas only within the boundaries of their competence, based on their education, training, supervised experience, consultation, study, or professional experience.

(b) Where scientific or professional knowledge in the discipline of psychology establishes that an understanding of factors associated with age, gender, gender identity, race, ethnicity, culture, national origin, religion, sexual orientation, disability, language, or socioeconomic status is essential for effective implementation of their services or research, psychologists have or obtain the training, experience, consultation, or supervision necessary to ensure the competence of their services, or they make appropriate referrals, except as provided in Standard 2.02, Providing Services in Emergencies.

(c) Psychologists planning to provide services, teach, or conduct research involving populations, areas, techniques, or technologies new to them undertake relevant education, training, supervised experience, consultation, or study.

(d) When psychologists are asked to provide services to individuals for whom appropriate mental health services are not available and for which psychologists have not obtained the competence necessary, psychologists with closely related prior training or experience may provide such services in order to ensure that services are not denied if they make a reasonable effort to obtain the competence required by using relevant research, training, consultation, or study.

(e) In those emerging areas in which generally recognized standards for preparatory training do not yet exist, psychologists nevertheless take reasonable steps to ensure the competence of their work and to protect clients/patients, students, supervisees, research participants, organizational clients, and others from harm.

(f) When assuming forensic roles, psychologists are or become reasonably familiar with the judicial or administrative rules governing their roles.

2.02 Providing Services in Emergencies

In emergencies, when psychologists provide services to individuals for whom other mental health services are not available and for which psychologists have not obtained the necessary training, psychologists may provide such services in order to ensure that services are not denied. The services are discontinued as soon as the emergency has ended or appropriate services are available.

2.03 Maintaining Competence

Psychologists undertake ongoing efforts to develop and maintain their competence.

2.04 Bases for Scientific and Professional Judgments

Psychologists' work is based upon established scientific and professional knowledge of the discipline. (See also Standards 2.01e, Boundaries of Competence, and 10.01b, Informed Consent to Therapy.)

2.05 Delegation of Work to Others

Psychologists who delegate work to employees, supervisees, or research or teaching assistants or who use the services of others, such as interpreters, take reasonable steps to (1) avoid delegating such work to persons who have a multiple relationship with those being served that would likely lead to exploitation or loss of objectivity; (2) authorize only those responsibilities that such persons can be expected to perform competently on the basis of their education, training, or experience, either independently or with the level of supervision being provided; and (3) see that such persons perform these services competently. (See also Standards 2.02, Providing Services in Emergencies; 3.05, Multiple Relationships; 4.01, Maintaining Confidentiality; 9.01, Bases for Assessments; 9.02, Use of Assessments; 9.03, Informed Consent in Assessments; and 9.07, Assessment by Unqualified Persons.)

2.06 Personal Problems and Conflicts

(a) Psychologists refrain from initiating an activity when they know or should know that there is a substantial likelihood that their personal problems will prevent them from performing their work-related activities in a competent manner.

(b) When psychologists become aware of personal problems that may interfere with their performing work-related duties adequately, they take appropriate measures, such as obtaining professional consultation or assistance, and determine whether they should limit, suspend, or terminate their work-related duties. (See also Standard 10.10, Terminating Therapy.)

3. HUMAN RELATIONS

3.01 Unfair Discrimination

In their work-related activities, psychologists do not engage in unfair discrimination based on age, gender, gender identity, race, ethnicity, culture, national origin, religion, sexual orientation, disability, socioeconomic status, or any basis proscribed by law.

3.02 Sexual Harassment

Psychologists do not engage in sexual harassment. Sexual harassment is sexual solicitation, physical advances, or verbal or nonverbal conduct that is sexual in nature, that occurs in connection with the psychologist's activities or roles as a psychologist, and that either (1) is unwelcome, is offensive, or creates a hostile workplace or educational environment, and the psychologist knows or is told this or (2) is sufficiently severe or intense to be abusive to a reasonable person in the context. Sexual harassment can consist of a single intense or severe act or of multiple persistent or pervasive acts. (See also Standard 1.08, Unfair Discrimination Against Complainants and Respondents.)

3.03 Other Harassment

Psychologists do not knowingly engage in behavior that is harassing or demeaning to persons with whom they interact in their work based on factors such as those persons' age, gender, gender identity, race, ethnicity, culture, national origin, religion, sexual orientation, disability, language, or socioeconomic status.

3.04 Avoiding Harm

Psychologists take reasonable steps to avoid harming their clients/patients, students, supervisees, research participants, organizational clients, and others with whom they work, and to minimize harm where it is foreseeable and unavoidable.

3.05 Multiple Relationships

(a) A multiple relationship occurs when a psychologist is in a professional role with a person and (1) at the same time is in another role with the same person, (2) at the same time is in a relationship with a person closely associated with or related to the person with whom the psychologist has the professional relationship, or (3) promises to enter into another relationship in the future with the person or a person closely associated with or related to the person.

A psychologist refrains from entering into a multiple relationship if the multiple relationship could reasonably be expected to impair the psychologist's objectivity, competence, or effectiveness in performing his or her functions as a psychologist, or otherwise risks exploitation or harm to the person with whom the professional relationship exists.

Multiple relationships that would not reasonably be expected to cause impairment or risk exploitation or harm are not unethical.

(b) If a psychologist finds that, due to unforeseen factors, a potentially harmful multiple relationship has arisen, the psychologist takes reasonable steps to resolve it with due regard for the best interests of the affected person and maximal compliance with the Ethics Code.

(c) When psychologists are required by law, institutional policy, or extraordinary circumstances to serve in more than one role in judicial or administrative proceedings, at the outset they clarify role expectations and the extent of confidentiality and thereafter as changes occur. (See also Standards 3.04, Avoiding Harm, and 3.07, Third-Party Requests for Services.)

3.06 Conflict of Interest

Psychologists refrain from taking on a professional role when personal, scientific, professional, legal, financial, or other interests or relationships could reasonably be expected to (1) impair their objectivity, competence, or effectiveness in performing their functions as psychologists or (2) expose the person or organization with whom the professional relationship exists to harm or exploitation.

3.07 Third-Party Requests for Services

When psychologists agree to provide services to a person or entity at the request of a third party, psychologists attempt to clarify at the outset of the service the nature of the relationship with all individuals or organizations involved. This clarification includes the role of the psychologist (e.g., therapist, consultant, diagnostician, or expert witness), an identification of who is the client, the probable uses of the services provided or the information obtained, and the fact that there may be limits to confidentiality. (See also Standards 3.05, Multiple Relationships, and 4.02, Discussing the Limits of Confidentiality.)

3.08 Exploitative Relationships

Psychologists do not exploit persons over whom they have supervisory, evaluative, or other authority such as clients/patients, students, supervisees, research participants, and employees. (See also Standards 3.05, Multiple Relationships; 6.04, Fees and Financial Arrangements; 6.05, Barter With Clients/Patients; 7.07, Sexual Relationships With Students and Supervisees; 10.05, Sexual Intimacies With Current Therapy Clients/Patients; 10.06, Sexual Intimacies With Relatives or Significant Others of Current Therapy Clients/Patients; 10.07, Therapy With Former Sexual Partners; and 10.08, Sexual Intimacies With Former Therapy Clients/Patients.)

3.09 Cooperation With Other Professionals

When indicated and professionally appropriate, psychologists cooperate with other professionals in order to serve their clients/patients effectively and appropriately. (See also Standard 4.05, Disclosures.)

3.10 Informed Consent

(a) When psychologists conduct research or provide assessment, therapy, counseling, or consulting services in person or via electronic transmission or other forms of communication, they obtain the informed consent of the individual or individuals using language that is reasonably understandable to that person or persons except when conducting such activities without consent is mandated by law or governmental regulation or as otherwise provided in this Ethics Code. (See also Standards 8.02, Informed Consent to Research; 9.03, Informed Consent in Assessments; and 10.01, Informed Consent to Therapy.)

(b) For persons who are legally incapable of giving informed consent, psychologists nevertheless (1) provide an appropriate explanation, (2) seek the individual's assent, (3) consider such persons' preferences and best interests, and (4) obtain appropriate permission from a legally authorized person, if such substitute consent is permitted or required by law. When consent by a legally authorized person is not permitted or required by law, psychologists take reasonable steps to protect the individual's rights and welfare.

(c) When psychological services are court ordered or otherwise mandated, psychologists inform the individual of the nature of the anticipated services, including whether the services are court ordered or mandated and any limits of confidentiality, before proceeding.

(d) Psychologists appropriately document written or oral consent, permission, and assent. (See also Standards 8.02, Informed Consent to Research; 9.03, Informed Consent in Assessments; and 10.01, Informed Consent to Therapy.)

3.11 Psychological Services Delivered To or Through Organizations

(a) Psychologists delivering services to or through organizations provide information beforehand to clients and when appropriate those directly affected by the services about (1) the nature and objectives of the services, (2) the intended recipients, (3) which of the individuals are clients, (4) the relationship the psychologist will have with each person and the organization, (5) the probable uses of services provided and information obtained, (6) who will have access to the information, and (7) limits of confidentiality. As soon as feasible, they provide information about the results and conclusions of such services to appropriate persons.

(b) If psychologists will be precluded by law or by organizational roles from providing such information to particular individuals or groups, they so inform those individuals or groups at the outset of the service.

3.12 Interruption of Psychological Services

Unless otherwise covered by contract, psychologists make reasonable efforts to plan for facilitating services in the event that psychological services are interrupted by factors such as the psychologist's illness, death, unavailability, relocation, or retirement or by the client's/patient's relocation or financial limitations. (See also Standard 6.02c, Maintenance, Dissemination, and Disposal of Confidential Records of Professional and Scientific Work.)

4. PRIVACY AND CONFIDENTIALITY

4.01 Maintaining Confidentiality

Psychologists have a primary obligation and take reasonable precautions to protect confidential information obtained through or stored in any medium, recognizing that the extent and limits of confidentiality may be regulated by law or established by institutional rules or professional or scientific relationship. (See also Standard 2.05, Delegation of Work to Others.)

4.02 Discussing the Limits of Confidentiality

(a) Psychologists discuss with persons (including, to the extent feasible, persons who are legally incapable of giving informed consent and their legal representatives) and organizations with whom they establish a scientific or professional relationship (1) the relevant limits of confidentiality and (2) the foreseeable uses of the information generated through their psychological activities. (See also Standard 3.10, Informed Consent.)

(b) Unless it is not feasible or is contraindicated, the discussion of confidentiality occurs at the outset of the relationship and thereafter as new circumstances may warrant.

(c) Psychologists who offer services, products, or information via electronic transmission inform clients/patients of the risks to privacy and limits of confidentiality.

4.03 Recording

Before recording the voices or images of individuals to whom they provide services, psychologists obtain permission from all such persons or their legal representatives. (See also Standards 8.03, Informed Consent for Recording Voices and Images in Research; 8.05, Dispensing With Informed Consent for Research; and 8.07, Deception in Research.)

4.04 Minimizing Intrusions on Privacy

(a) Psychologists include in written and oral reports and consultations, only information germane to the purpose for which the communication is made.
(b) Psychologists discuss confidential information obtained in their work only for appropriate scientific or professional purposes and only with persons clearly concerned with such matters.

4.05 Disclosures

(a) Psychologists may disclose confidential information with the appropriate consent of the organizational client, the individual client/patient, or another legally authorized person on behalf of the client/patient unless prohibited by law.
(b) Psychologists disclose confidential information without the consent of the individual only as mandated by law, or where permitted by law for a valid purpose such as to (1) provide needed professional services; (2) obtain appropriate professional consultations; (3) protect the client/patient, psychologist, or others from harm; or (4) obtain payment for services from a client/patient, in which instance disclosure is limited to the minimum that is necessary to achieve the purpose. (See also Standard 6.04e, Fees and Financial Arrangements.)

4.06 Consultations

When consulting with colleagues, (1) psychologists do not disclose confidential information that reasonably could lead to the identification of a client/patient, research participant, or other person or organization with whom they have a confidential relationship unless they have obtained the prior consent of the person or organization or the disclosure cannot be avoided, and (2) they disclose information only to the extent necessary to achieve the purposes of the consultation. (See also Standard 4.01, Maintaining Confidentiality.)

4.07 Use of Confidential Information for Didactic or Other Purposes

Psychologists do not disclose in their writings, lectures, or other public media, confidential, personally identifiable information concerning their clients/patients, students, research participants, organizational clients, or other recipients of their services that they obtained during the course of their work, unless (1) they take reasonable steps to disguise the person or organization, (2) the person or organization has consented in writing, or (3) there is legal authorization for doing so.

5. ADVERTISING AND OTHER PUBLIC STATEMENTS

5.01 Avoidance of False or Deceptive Statements

(a) Public statements include but are not limited to paid or unpaid advertising, product endorsements, grant applications, licensing applications, other credentialing applications, brochures, printed matter, directory listings, personal resumes or curricula vitae, or comments for use in media such as print or electronic transmission, statements in legal proceedings, lectures and public oral presentations, and published materials. Psychologists do not knowingly make public statements that are false, deceptive, or fraudulent concerning their research, practice, or other work activities or those of persons or organizations with which they are affiliated.

(b) Psychologists do not make false, deceptive, or fraudulent statements concerning (1) their training, experience, or competence; (2) their academic degrees; (3) their credentials; (4) their institutional or association affiliations; (5) their services; (6) the scientific or clinical basis for, or results or degree of success of, their services; (7) their fees; or (8) their publications or research findings.

(c) Psychologists claim degrees as credentials for their health services only if those degrees (1) were earned from a regionally accredited educational institution or (2) were the basis for psychology licensure by the state in which they practice.

5.02 Statements by Others

(a) Psychologists who engage others to create or place public statements that promote their professional practice, products, or activities retain professional responsibility for such statements.

(b) Psychologists do not compensate employees of press, radio, television, or other communication media in return for publicity in a news item. (See also Standard 1.01, Misuse of Psychologists' Work.)

(c) A paid advertisement relating to psychologists' activities must be identified or clearly recognizable as such.

5.03 Descriptions of Workshops and Non-Degree-Granting Educational Programs

To the degree to which they exercise control, psychologists responsible for announcements, catalogs, brochures, or advertisements describing workshops, seminars, or other non-degree-granting educational programs ensure that they accurately describe the audience for which the program is intended, the educational objectives, the presenters, and the fees involved.

5.04 Media Presentations

When psychologists provide public advice or comment via print, internet, or other electronic transmission, they take precautions to ensure that statements (1) are based on their professional knowledge, training, or experience in accord with appropriate psychological literature and practice; (2) are otherwise consistent with this Ethics Code; and (3) do not indicate that a professional relationship has been established with the recipient. (See also Standard 2.04, Bases for Scientific and Professional Judgments.)

5.05 Testimonials

Psychologists do not solicit testimonials from current therapy clients/patients or other persons who because of their particular circumstances are vulnerable to undue influence.

5.06 In-Person Solicitation

Psychologists do not engage, directly or through agents, in uninvited in-person solicitation of business from actual or potential therapy clients/patients or other persons who because of their particular circumstances are vulnerable to undue influence. However, this prohibition does not preclude (1) attempting to implement appropriate collateral contacts for the purpose of benefiting an already engaged therapy client/patient or (2) providing disaster or community outreach services.

6. RECORD KEEPING AND FEES

6.01 Documentation of Professional and Scientific Work and Maintenance of Records

Psychologists create, and to the extent the records are under their control, maintain, disseminate, store, retain, and dispose of records and data relating to their professional and scientific work in order to (1) facilitate provision of services later by them or by other professionals, (2) allow for replication of research design and analyses, (3) meet institutional requirements, (4) ensure accuracy of billing and payments, and (5) ensure compliance with law. (See also Standard 4.01, Maintaining Confidentiality.)

6.02 Maintenance, Dissemination, and Disposal of Confidential Records of Professional and Scientific Work

(a) Psychologists maintain confidentiality in creating, storing, accessing, transferring, and disposing of records under their control, whether these are written, automated, or in any other medium. (See also Standards 4.01, Maintaining Confidentiality, and 6.01, Documentation of Professional and Scientific Work and Maintenance of Records.)

(b) If confidential information concerning recipients of psychological services is entered into databases or systems of records available to persons whose access has not been consented to by the recipient, psychologists use coding or other techniques to avoid the inclusion of personal identifiers.

(c) Psychologists make plans in advance to facilitate the appropriate transfer and to protect the confidentiality of records and data in the event of psychologists' withdrawal from positions or practice. (See also Standards 3.12, Interruption of Psychological Services, and 10.09, Interruption of Therapy.)

6.03 Withholding Records for Nonpayment

Psychologists may not withhold records under their control that are requested and needed for a client's/patient's emergency treatment solely because payment has not been received.

6.04 Fees and Financial Arrangements

(a) As early as is feasible in a professional or scientific relationship, psychologists and recipients of psychological services reach an agreement specifying compensation and billing arrangements.
(b) Psychologists' fee practices are consistent with law.
(c) Psychologists do not misrepresent their fees.
(d) If limitations to services can be anticipated because of limitations in financing, this is discussed with the recipient of services as early as is feasible. (See also Standards 10.09, Interruption of Therapy, and 10.10, Terminating Therapy.)
(e) If the recipient of services does not pay for services as agreed, and if psychologists intend to use collection agencies or legal measures to collect the fees, psychologists first inform the person that such measures will be taken and provide that person an opportunity to make prompt payment. (See also Standards 4.05, Disclosures; 6.03, Withholding Records for Nonpayment; and 10.01, Informed Consent to Therapy.)

6.05 Barter With Clients/Patients

Barter is the acceptance of goods, services, or other nonmonetary remuneration from clients/patients in return for psychological services. Psychologists may barter only if (1) it is not clinically contraindicated, and (2) the resulting arrangement is not exploitative. (See also Standards 3.05, Multiple Relationships, and 6.04, Fees and Financial Arrangements.)

6.06 Accuracy in Reports to Payors and Funding Sources

In their reports to payors for services or sources of research funding, psychologists take reasonable steps to ensure the accurate reporting of the nature of the service provided or research conducted, the fees, charges, or payments, and where applicable, the identity of the provider, the findings, and the diagnosis. (See also Standards 4.01, Maintaining Confidentiality; 4.04, Minimizing Intrusions on Privacy; and 4.05, Disclosures.)

6.07 Referrals and Fees

When psychologists pay, receive payment from, or divide fees with another professional, other than in an employer-employee relationship, the payment to each is based on the services provided (clinical, consultative, administrative, or other) and is not based on the referral itself. (See also Standard 3.09, Cooperation With Other Professionals.)

7. EDUCATION AND TRAINING

7.01 Design of Education and Training Programs

Psychologists responsible for education and training programs take reasonable steps to ensure that the programs are designed to provide the appropriate knowledge and proper experiences, and to meet the requirements for licensure, certification, or other goals for which claims are made by the program. (See also Standard 5.03, Descriptions of Workshops and Non-Degree-Granting Educational Programs.)

7.02 Descriptions of Education and Training Programs

Psychologists responsible for education and training programs take reasonable steps to ensure that there is a current and accurate description of the program content (including participation in required course- or program-related counseling, psychotherapy, experiential groups, consulting projects, or community service), training goals and objectives, stipends and benefits, and requirements that must be met for satisfactory completion of the program. This information must be made readily available to all interested parties.

7.03 Accuracy in Teaching

(a) Psychologists take reasonable steps to ensure that course syllabi are accurate regarding the subject matter to be covered, bases for evaluating progress, and the nature of course experiences. This standard does not preclude an instructor from modifying course content or requirements when the instructor considers it pedagogically necessary or desirable, so long as students are made aware of these modifications in a manner that enables them to fulfill course requirements. (See also Standard 5.01, Avoidance of False or Deceptive Statements.)

(b) When engaged in teaching or training, psychologists present psychological information accurately. (See also Standard 2.03, Maintaining Competence.)

7.04 Student Disclosure of Personal Information

Psychologists do not require students or supervisees to disclose personal information in course- or program-related activities, either orally or in writing, regarding sexual history, history of abuse and neglect, psychological treatment, and relationships with parents, peers, and spouses or significant others except if (1) the program or training facility has clearly identified this requirement in its admissions and program materials or (2) the information is necessary to evaluate or obtain assistance for students whose personal problems could reasonably be judged to be preventing them from performing their training- or professionally related activities in a competent manner or posing a threat to the students or others.

7.05 Mandatory Individual or Group Therapy

(a) When individual or group therapy is a program or course requirement, psychologists responsible for that program allow students in undergraduate and graduate programs the option of selecting such therapy from practitioners unaffiliated with the program. (See also Standard 7.02, Descriptions of Education and Training Programs.)

(b) Faculty who are or are likely to be responsible for evaluating students' academic performance do not themselves provide that therapy. (See also Standard 3.05, Multiple Relationships.)

7.06 Assessing Student and Supervisee Performance

(a) In academic and supervisory relationships, psychologists establish a timely and specific process for providing feedback to students and supervisees. Information regarding the process is provided to the student at the beginning of supervision.

(b) Psychologists evaluate students and supervisees on the basis of their actual performance on relevant and established program requirements.

7.07 Sexual Relationships With Students and Supervisees

Psychologists do not engage in sexual relationships with students or supervisees who are in their department, agency, or training center or over whom psychologists have or are likely to have evaluative authority. (See also Standard 3.05, Multiple Relationships.)

8. RESEARCH AND PUBLICATION

8.01 Institutional Approval

When institutional approval is required, psychologists provide accurate information about their research proposals and obtain approval prior to conducting the research. They conduct the research in accordance with the approved research protocol.

8.02 Informed Consent to Research

(a) When obtaining informed consent as required in Standard 3.10, Informed Consent, psychologists inform participants about (1) the purpose of the research, expected duration, and procedures; (2) their right to decline to participate and to withdraw from the research once participation has begun; (3) the foreseeable consequences of declining or withdrawing; (4) reasonably foreseeable factors that may be expected to influence their willingness to participate such as potential risks, discomfort, or adverse effects; (5) any prospective research benefits; (6) limits of confidentiality; (7) incentives for participation; and (8) whom to contact for questions about the research and research participants' rights. They provide opportunity for the prospective participants to ask questions and receive answers. (See also Standards 8.03, Informed Consent for Recording Voices and Images in Research; 8.05, Dispensing With Informed Consent for Research; and 8.07, Deception in Research.)

(b) Psychologists conducting intervention research involving the use of experimental treatments clarify to participants at the outset of the research (1) the experimental nature of the treatment; (2) the services that will or will not be available to the control group(s) if appropriate; (3) the means by which assignment to treatment and control groups will be made; (4) available treatment alternatives if an individual does not wish to participate in the research or wishes to withdraw once a study has begun; and (5) compensation for or monetary costs of participating including, if appropriate, whether reimbursement from the participant or a third-party payor will be sought. (See also Standard 8.02a, Informed Consent to Research.)

8.03 Informed Consent for Recording Voices and Images in Research

Psychologists obtain informed consent from research participants prior to recording their voices or images for data collection unless (1) the research consists solely of naturalistic observations in public places, and it is not anticipated that the recording will be used in a manner that could cause personal identification or harm, or (2) the research design includes deception, and consent for the use of the recording is obtained during debriefing. (See also Standard 8.07, Deception in Research.)

8.04 Client/Patient, Student, and Subordinate Research Participants

(a) When psychologists conduct research with clients/patients, students, or subordinates as participants, psychologists take steps to protect the prospective participants from adverse consequences of declining or withdrawing from participation.

(b) When research participation is a course requirement or an opportunity for extra credit, the prospective participant is given the choice of equitable alternative activities.

8.05 Dispensing With Informed Consent for Research

Psychologists may dispense with informed consent only (1) where research would not reasonably be assumed to create distress or harm and involves (a) the study of normal educational practices, curricula, or classroom management methods conducted in educational settings; (b) only anonymous questionnaires, naturalistic observations, or archival research

for which disclosure of responses would not place participants at risk of criminal or civil liability or damage their financial standing, employability, or reputation, and confidentiality is protected; or (c) the study of factors related to job or
organization effectiveness conducted in organizational settings
for which there is no risk to participants' employability, and
confidentiality is protected or (2) where otherwise permitted
by law or federal or institutional regulations.

8.06 Offering Inducements for Research Participation

(a) Psychologists make reasonable efforts to avoid offering
excessive or inappropriate financial or other inducements
for research participation when such inducements are
likely to coerce participation.

(b) When offering professional services as an inducement for
research participation, psychologists clarify the nature of
the services, as well as the risks, obligations, and limitations. (See also Standard 6.05, Barter With Clients/Pa-
tients.)

8.07 Deception in Research

(a) Psychologists do not conduct a study involving deception
unless they have determined that the use of deceptive techniques is justified by the study's significant prospective
scientific, educational, or applied value and that effective
nondeceptive alternative procedures are not feasible.

(b) Psychologists do not deceive prospective participants about
research that is reasonably expected to cause physical pain
or severe emotional distress.

(c) Psychologists explain any deception that is an integral feature of the design and conduct of an experiment to participants as early as is feasible, preferably at the conclusion
of their participation, but no later than at the conclusion
of the data collection, and permit participants to withdraw
their data. (See also Standard 8.08, Debriefing.)

8.08 Debriefing

(a) Psychologists provide a prompt opportunity for participants to obtain appropriate information about the nature,
results, and conclusions of the research, and they take rea-

sonable steps to correct any misconceptions that participants may have of which the psychologists are aware.

(b) If scientific or humane values justify delaying or withholding this information, psychologists take reasonable measures to reduce the risk of harm.

(c) When psychologists become aware that research procedures have harmed a participant, they take reasonable steps to minimize the harm.

8.09 Humane Care and Use of Animals in Research

(a) Psychologists acquire, care for, use, and dispose of animals in compliance with current federal, state, and local laws and regulations, and with professional standards.

(b) Psychologists trained in research methods and experienced in the care of laboratory animals supervise all procedures involving animals and are responsible for ensuring appropriate consideration of their comfort, health, and humane treatment.

(c) Psychologists ensure that all individuals under their supervision who are using animals have received instruction in research methods and in the care, maintenance, and handling of the species being used, to the extent appropriate to their role. (See also Standard 2.05, Delegation of Work to Others.)

(d) Psychologists make reasonable efforts to minimize the discomfort, infection, illness, and pain of animal subjects.

(e) Psychologists use a procedure subjecting animals to pain, stress, or privation only when an alternative procedure is unavailable and the goal is justified by its prospective scientific, educational, or applied value.

(f) Psychologists perform surgical procedures under appropriate anesthesia and follow techniques to avoid infection and minimize pain during and after surgery.

(g) When it is appropriate that an animal's life be terminated, psychologists proceed rapidly, with an effort to minimize pain and in accordance with accepted procedures.

8.10 Reporting Research Results

(a) Psychologists do not fabricate data. (See also Standard 5.01a, Avoidance of False or Deceptive Statements.)

(b) If psychologists discover significant errors in their published data, they take reasonable steps to correct such errors in a correction, retraction, erratum, or other appropriate publication means.

8.11 Plagiarism

Psychologists do not present portions of another's work or data as their own, even if the other work or data source is cited occasionally.

8.12 Publication Credit

(a) Psychologists take responsibility and credit, including authorship credit, only for work they have actually performed or to which they have substantially contributed. (See also Standard 8.12b, Publication Credit.)

(b) Principal authorship and other publication credits accurately reflect the relative scientific or professional contributions of the individuals involved, regardless of their relative status. Mere possession of an institutional position, such as department chair, does not justify authorship credit. Minor contributions to the research or to the writing for publications are acknowledged appropriately, such as in footnotes or in an introductory statement.

(c) Except under exceptional circumstances, a student is listed as principal author on any multiple-authored article that is substantially based on the student's doctoral dissertation. Faculty advisors discuss publication credit with students as early as feasible and throughout the research and publication process as appropriate. (See also Standard 8.12b, Publication Credit.)

8.13 Duplicate Publication of Data

Psychologists do not publish, as original data, data that have been previously published. This does not preclude republishing data when they are accompanied by proper acknowledgment.

8.14 Sharing Research Data for Verification

(a) After research results are published, psychologists do not withhold the data on which their conclusions are based from other competent professionals who seek to verify the substantive claims through reanalysis and who intend to use such data only for that purpose, provided that the confidentiality of the participants can be protected and unless legal rights concerning proprietary data preclude their release. This does not preclude psychologists from requiring that such individuals or groups be responsible for costs associated with the provision of such information.

(b) Psychologists who request data from other psychologists to verify the substantive claims through reanalysis may use shared data only for the declared purpose. Requesting psychologists obtain prior written agreement for all other uses of the data.

8.15 Reviewers

Psychologists who review material submitted for presentation, publication, grant, or research proposal review respect the confidentiality of and the proprietary rights in such information of those who submitted it.

9. ASSESSMENT

9.01 Bases for Assessments

(a) Psychologists base the opinions contained in their recommendations, reports, and diagnostic or evaluative statements, including forensic testimony, on information and techniques sufficient to substantiate their findings. (See also Standard 2.04, Bases for Scientific and Professional Judgments.)

(b) Except as noted in 9.01c, psychologists provide opinions of the psychological characteristics of individuals only after they have conducted an examination of the individuals adequate to support their statements or conclusions. When, despite reasonable efforts, such an examination is not practical, psychologists document the efforts they made and the result of those efforts, clarify the probable impact of their limited information on the reliability and validity of their opinions, and appropriately limit the nature and extent of their conclusions or recommendations. (See also Standards 2.01, Boundaries of Competence, and 9.06, Interpreting Assessment Results.)

(c) When psychologists conduct a record review or provide consultation or supervision and an individual examination is not warranted or necessary for the opinion, psychologists explain this and the sources of information on which they based their conclusions and recommendations.

9.02　Use of Assessments

(a) Psychologists administer, adapt, score, interpret, or use assessment techniques, interviews, tests, or instruments in a manner and for purposes that are appropriate in light of the research on or evidence of the usefulness and proper application of the techniques.

(b) Psychologists use assessment instruments whose validity and reliability have been established for use with members of the population tested. When such validity or reliability has not been established, psychologists describe the strengths and limitations of test results and interpretation.

(c) Psychologists use assessment methods that are appropriate to an individual's language preference and competence, unless the use of an alternative language is relevant to the assessment issues.

9.03　Informed Consent in Assessments

(a) Psychologists obtain informed consent for assessments, evaluations, or diagnostic services, as described in Standard 3.10, Informed Consent, except when (1) testing is mandated by law or governmental regulations; (2) informed consent is implied because testing is conducted as a routine educational, institutional, or organizational activity (e.g., when participants voluntarily agree to assessment when applying for a job); or (3) one purpose of the testing is to evaluate decisional capacity. Informed consent includes an explanation of the nature and purpose of the assessment, fees, involvement of third parties, and limits of confidentiality and sufficient opportunity for the client/patient to ask questions and receive answers.

(b) Psychologists inform persons with questionable capacity to consent or for whom testing is mandated by law or governmental regulations about the nature and purpose of the proposed assessment services, using language that is reasonably understandable to the person being assessed.

(c) Psychologists using the services of an interpreter obtain informed consent from the client/patient to use that interpreter, ensure that confidentiality of test results and test security are maintained, and include in their recommendations, reports, and diagnostic or evaluative statements, including forensic testimony, discussion of any limitations on the data obtained. (See also Standards 2.05, Delegation of Work to Others; 4.01, Maintaining Confidentiality; 9.01, Bases for Assessments; 9.06, Interpreting Assessment Results; and 9.07, Assessment by Unqualified Persons.)

9.04 Release of Test Data

(a) The term *test data* refers to raw and scaled scores, client/patient responses to test questions or stimuli, and psychologists' notes and recordings concerning client/patient statements and behavior during an examination. Those portions of test materials that include client/patient responses are included in the definition of *test data*. Pursuant to a client/patient release, psychologists provide test data to the client/patient or other persons identified in the release. Psychologists may refrain from releasing test data to protect a client/patient or others from substantial harm or misuse or misrepresentation of the data or the test, recognizing that in many instances release of confidential information under these circumstances is regulated by law. (See also Standard 9.11, Maintaining Test Security.)

(b) In the absence of a client/patient release, psychologists provide test data only as required by law or court order.

9.05 Test Construction

Psychologists who develop tests and other assessment techniques use appropriate psychometric procedures and current scientific or professional knowledge for test design, standardization, validation, reduction or elimination of bias, and recommendations for use.

9.06 Interpreting Assessment Results

When interpreting assessment results, including automated interpretations, psychologists take into account the purpose of the assessment as well as the various test factors, test-taking abilities, and other characteristics of the person being assessed, such as situational, personal, linguistic, and cultural differences, that might affect psychologists' judgments or reduce the accuracy of their interpretations. They indicate any significant limitations of their interpretations. (See also Standards 2.01b and c, Boundaries of Competence, and 3.01, Unfair Discrimination.)

9.07 Assessment by Unqualified Persons

Psychologists do not promote the use of psychological assessment techniques by unqualified persons, except when such use is conducted for training purposes with appropriate supervision. (See also Standard 2.05, Delegation of Work to Others.)

9.08 Obsolete Tests and Outdated Test Results

(a) Psychologists do not base their assessment or intervention decisions or recommendations on data or test results that are outdated for the current purpose.

(b) Psychologists do not base such decisions or recommendations on tests and measures that are obsolete and not useful for the current purpose.

9.09 Test Scoring and Interpretation Services

(a) Psychologists who offer assessment or scoring services to other professionals accurately describe the purpose, norms, validity, reliability, and applications of the procedures and any special qualifications applicable to their use.

(b) Psychologists select scoring and interpretation services (including automated services) on the basis of evidence of the validity of the program and procedures as well as on other appropriate considerations. (See also Standard 2.01b and c, Boundaries of Competence.)

(c) Psychologists retain responsibility for the appropriate application, interpretation, and use of assessment instruments, whether they score and interpret such tests themselves or use automated or other services.

9.10 Explaining Assessment Results

Regardless of whether the scoring and interpretation are done by psychologists, by employees or assistants, or by automated or other outside services, psychologists take reasonable steps to ensure that explanations of results are given to the individual or designated representative unless the nature of the relationship precludes provision of an explanation of results (such as in some organizational consulting, preemployment or security screenings, and forensic evaluations), and this fact has been clearly explained to the person being assessed in advance.

9.11 Maintaining Test Security

The term *test materials* refers to manuals, instruments, protocols, and test questions or stimuli and does not include *test data* as defined in Standard 9.04, Release of Test Data. Psychologists make reasonable efforts to maintain the integrity and security of test materials and other assessment techniques consistent with law and contractual obligations, and in a manner that permits adherence to this Ethics Code.

10. THERAPY

10.01 Informed Consent to Therapy

(a) When obtaining informed consent to therapy as required in Standard 3.10, Informed Consent, psychologists inform clients/patients as early as is feasible in the therapeutic relationship about the nature and anticipated course of therapy, fees, involvement of third parties, and limits of confidentiality and provide sufficient opportunity for the client/patient to ask questions and receive answers. (See also Standards 4.02, Discussing the Limits of Confidentiality, and 6.04, Fees and Financial Arrangements.)

(b) When obtaining informed consent for treatment for which generally recognized techniques and procedures have not been established, psychologists inform their clients/patients of the developing nature of the treatment, the potential risks involved, alternative treatments that may be available, and the voluntary nature of their participation. (See also Standards 2.01e, Boundaries of Competence, and 3.10, Informed Consent.)

(c) When the therapist is a trainee and the legal responsibility for the treatment provided resides with the supervisor, the client/patient, as part of the informed consent procedure, is informed that the therapist is in training and is being supervised and is given the name of the supervisor.

10.02 Therapy Involving Couples or Families

(a) When psychologists agree to provide services to several persons who have a relationship (such as spouses, significant others, or parents and children), they take reasonable steps to clarify at the outset (1) which of the individuals are clients/patients and (2) the relationship the psychologist will have with each person. This clarification includes the psychologist's role and the probable uses of the services provided or the information obtained. (See also Standard 4.02, Discussing the Limits of Confidentiality.)

(b) If it becomes apparent that psychologists may be called on to perform potentially conflicting roles (such as family therapist and then witness for one party in divorce proceedings), psychologists take reasonable steps to clarify and modify, or withdraw from, roles appropriately. (See also Standard 3.05c, Multiple Relationships.)

10.03 Group Therapy

When psychologists provide services to several persons in a group setting, they describe at the outset the roles and responsibilities of all parties and the limits of confidentiality.

10.04 Providing Therapy to Those Served by Others

In deciding whether to offer or provide services to those already receiving mental health services elsewhere, psychologists carefully consider the treatment issues and the potential client's/patient's welfare. Psychologists discuss these issues with the client/patient or another legally authorized person on behalf of the client/patient in order to minimize the risk of confusion and conflict, consult with the other service providers when appropriate, and proceed with caution and sensitivity to the therapeutic issues.

10.05 Sexual Intimacies With Current Therapy Clients/Patients

Psychologists do not engage in sexual intimacies with current therapy clients/patients.

10.06 Sexual Intimacies With Relatives or Significant Others of Current Therapy Clients/Patients

Psychologists do not engage in sexual intimacies with individuals they know to be close relatives, guardians, or significant others of current clients/patients. Psychologists do not terminate therapy to circumvent this standard.

10.07 Therapy With Former Sexual Partners

Psychologists do not accept as therapy clients/patients persons with whom they have engaged in sexual intimacies.

10.08 Sexual Intimacies With Former Therapy Clients/Patients

(a) Psychologists do not engage in sexual intimacies with former clients/patients for at least two years after cessation or termination of therapy.

(b) Psychologists do not engage in sexual intimacies with former clients/patients even after a two-year interval except in the most unusual circumstances. Psychologists who engage in such activity after the two years following cessation or termination of therapy and of having no sexual contact with the former client/patient bear the burden of demonstrating that there has been no exploitation, in light of all relevant factors, including (1) the amount of time that has passed since therapy terminated; (2) the nature, duration, and intensity of the therapy; (3) the circumstances of termination; (4) the client's/patient's personal history; (5) the client's/patient's current mental status; (6) the likelihood of adverse impact on the client/patient; and (7) any statements or actions made by the therapist during the course of therapy suggesting or inviting the possibility of a posttermination sexual or romantic relationship with the client/patient. (See also Standard 3.05, Multiple Relationships.)

10.09 Interruption of Therapy

When entering into employment or contractual relationships, psychologists make reasonable efforts to provide for orderly and appropriate resolution of responsibility for client/patient care in the event that the employment or contractual relationship ends, with paramount consideration given to the welfare of the client/patient. (See also Standard 3.12, Interruption of Psychological Services.)

10.10 Terminating Therapy

    (a) Psychologists terminate therapy when it becomes reasonably clear that the client/patient no longer needs the service, is not likely to benefit, or is being harmed by continued service.

    (b) Psychologists may terminate therapy when threatened or otherwise endangered by the client/patient or another person with whom the client/patient has a relationship.

    (c) Except where precluded by the actions of clients/patients or third-party payors, prior to termination psychologists provide pretermination counseling and suggest alternative service providers as appropriate.

Appendix E

CODE OF ETHICS
National Association of
Social Workers (NASW)*

PREAMBLE

The primary mission of the social work profession is to enhance human well-being and help meet the basic human needs of all people, with particular attention to the needs and empowerment of people who are vulnerable, oppressed, and living in poverty. A historic and defining feature of social work is the profession's focus on individual well-being in a social context and the well-being of society. Fundamental to social work is attention to the environmental forces that create, contribute to, and address problems in living.

Social workers promote social justice and social change with and on behalf of clients. "Clients" is used inclusively to refer to individuals, families, groups, organizations, and communities. Social workers are sensitive to cultural and ethnic diversity and strive to end discrimination, oppression, poverty, and other forms of social injustice. These activities may be in the form of direct practice, community organizing, supervision, consultation, administration, advocacy, social and political action, policy development and implementation, education, and research and evaluation. Social workers seek to enhance the capacity of people to address their own needs. Social workers also seek to promote the respon-

*From *Code of Ethics of the National Association of Social Workers (NASW)*. Copyright © 1999 by the National Association of Social Workers, Inc. Approved by the 1996 NASW Delegate Assembly and revised by the 1999 NASW Delegate Assembly. Reprinted with permission.

siveness of organizations, communities, and other social institutions to individuals' needs and social problems.

The mission of the social work profession is rooted in a set of core values. These core values, embraced by social workers throughout the profession's history, are the foundation of social work's unique purpose and perspective:

- service
- social justice
- dignity and worth of the person
- importance of human relationships
- integrity
- competence

This constellation of core values reflects what is unique to the social work profession. Core values, and the principles that flow from them, must be balanced within the context and complexity of the human experience.

Purpose of the NASW Code of Ethics

Professional ethics are at the core of social work. The profession has an obligation to articulate its basic values, ethical principles, and ethical standards. The *NASW Code of Ethics* sets forth these values, principles, and standards to guide social workers' conduct. The *Code* is relevant to all social workers and social work students, regardless of their professional functions, the settings in which they work, or the populations they serve.

The *NASW Code of Ethics* serves six purposes:

1. The *Code* identifies core values on which social work's mission is based.
2. The *Code* summarizes broad ethical principles that reflect the profession's core values and establishes a set of specific ethical standards that should be used to guide social work practice.
3. The *Code* is designed to help social workers identify relevant considerations when professional obligations conflict or ethical uncertainties arise.
4. The *Code* provides ethical standards to which the general public can hold the social work profession accountable.
5. The *Code* socializes practitioners new to the field to social work's mission, values, ethical principles, and ethical standards.

6. The *Code* articulates standards that the social work profession itself can use to assess whether social workers have engaged in unethical conduct. NASW has formal procedures to adjudicate ethics complaints filed against its members.* In subscribing to this *Code,* social workers are required to cooperate in its implementation, participate in NASW adjudication proceedings, and abide by any NASW disciplinary rulings or sanctions based on it.

The *Code* offers a set of values, principles, and standards to guide decision making and conduct when ethical issues arise. It does not provide a set of rules that prescribe how social workers should act in all situations. Specific applications of the *Code* must take into account the context in which it is being considered and the possibility of conflicts among the *Code's* values, principles, and standards. Ethical responsibilities flow from all human relationships, from the personal and familial to the social and professional.

Further, the *NASW Code of Ethics* does not specify which values, principles, and standards are most important and ought to outweigh others in instances when they conflict. Reasonable differences of opinion can and do exist among social workers with respect to the ways in which values, ethical principles, and ethical standards should be rank ordered when they conflict. Ethical decision making in a given situation must apply the informed judgment of the individual social worker and should also consider how the issues would be judged in a peer review process where the ethical standards of the profession would be applied.

Ethical decision making is a process. There are many instances in social work where simple answers are not available to resolve complex ethical issues. Social workers should take into consideration all the values, principles, and standards in this *Code* that are relevant to any situation in which ethical judgment is warranted. Social workers' decisions and actions should be consistent with the spirit as well as the letter of this *Code.*

In addition to this *Code,* there are many other sources of information about ethical thinking that may be useful. Social workers should consider ethical theory and principles generally, social work theory and research, laws, regulations, agency policies, and other relevant codes of ethics, recognizing that among codes of ethics social workers should consider the

---

*For information on NASW adjudication procedures, see *NASW Procedures for the Adjudication of Grievances.*

NASW Code of Ethics as their primary source. Social workers also should be aware of the impact on ethical decision making of their clients' and their own personal values and cultural and religious beliefs and practices. They should be aware of any conflicts between personal and professional values and deal with them responsibly. For additional guidance social workers should consult the relevant literature on professional ethics and ethical decision making and seek appropriate consultation when faced with ethical dilemmas. This may involve consultation with an agency-based or social work organization's ethics committee, a regulatory body, knowledgeable colleagues, supervisors, or legal counsel.

Instances may arise when social workers' ethical obligations conflict with agency policies or relevant laws or regulations. When such conflicts occur, social workers must make a responsible effort to resolve the conflict in a manner that is consistent with the values, principles, and standards expressed in this *Code*. If a reasonable resolution of the conflict does not appear possible, social workers should seek proper consultation before making a decision.

The *NASW Code of Ethics* is to be used by NASW and by individuals, agencies, organizations, and bodies (such as licensing and regulatory boards, professional liability insurance providers, courts of law, agency boards of directors, government agencies, and other professional groups) that choose to adopt it or use it as a frame of reference. Violation of standards in this *Code* does not automatically imply legal liability or violation of the law. Such determination can only be made in the context of legal and judicial proceedings. Alleged violations of the *Code* would be subject to a peer review process. Such processes are generally separate from legal or administrative procedures and insulated from legal review or proceedings to allow the profession to counsel and discipline its own members.

A code of ethics cannot guarantee ethical behavior. Moreover, a code of ethics cannot resolve all ethical issues or disputes or capture the richness and complexity involved in striving to make responsible choices within a moral community. Rather, a code of ethics sets forth values, ethical principles, and ethical standards to which professionals aspire and by which their actions can be judged. Social workers' ethical behavior should result from their personal commitment to engage in ethical practice. The *NASW Code of Ethics* reflects the commitment of all social workers to uphold the profession's values and to act ethically. Principles and standards must be applied by individuals of good character who discern moral questions and, in good faith, seek to make reliable ethical judgments.

ETHICAL PRINCIPLES

The following broad ethical principles are based on social work's core values of service, social justice, dignity and worth of the person, importance of human relationships, integrity, and competence. These principles set forth ideals to which all social workers should aspire.

Value: *Service*
Ethical Principle: *Social workers' primary goal is to help people in need and to address social problems.*

Social workers elevate service to others above self-interest. Social workers draw on their knowledge, values, and skills to help people in need and to address social problems. Social workers are encouraged to volunteer some portion of their professional skills with no expectation of significant financial return (pro bono service).

Value: *Social Justice*
Ethical Principle: *Social workers challenge social injustice.*

Social workers pursue social change, particularly with and on behalf of vulnerable and oppressed individuals and groups of people. Social workers' social change efforts are focused primarily on issues of poverty, unemployment, discrimination, and other forms of social injustice. These activities seek to promote sensitivity to and knowledge about oppression and cultural and ethnic diversity. Social workers strive to ensure access to needed information, services, and resources; equality of opportunity; and meaningful participation in decision making for all people.

Value: *Dignity and Worth of the Person*
Ethical Principle: *Social workers respect the inherent dignity and worth of the person.*

Social workers treat each person in a caring and respectful fashion, mindful of individual differences and cultural and ethnic diversity. Social workers promote clients' socially responsible self-determination. Social workers seek to enhance clients' capacity and opportunity to change and to address their own needs. Social workers are cognizant of their dual responsibility to clients and to the broader society. They seek to resolve conflicts between clients' interests and the broader society's interests in a socially responsible manner consistent with the values, ethical principles, and ethical standards of the profession.

Value: *Importance of Human Relationships*
Ethical Principle: *Social workers recognize the central importance of human relationships.*

Social workers understand that relationships between and among people are an important vehicle for change. Social workers engage people as partners in the helping process. Social workers seek to strengthen relationships among people in a purposeful effort to promote, restore, maintain, and enhance the well-being of individuals, families, social groups, organizations, and communities.

Value: *Integrity*
Ethical Principle: *Social workers behave in a trustworthy manner.*

Social workers are continually aware of the profession's mission, values, ethical principles, and ethical standards and practice in a manner consistent with them. Social workers act honestly and responsibly and promote ethical practices on the part of the organizations with which they are affiliated.

Value: *Competence*
Ethical Principle: *Social workers practice within their areas of competence and develop and enhance their professional expertise.*

Social workers continually strive to increase their professional knowledge and skills and to apply them in practice. Social workers should aspire to contribute to the knowledge base of the profession.

ETHICAL STANDARDS

The following ethical standards are relevant to the professional activities of all social workers. These standards concern (1) social workers' ethical responsibilities to clients, (2) social workers' ethical responsibilities to colleagues, (3) social workers' ethical responsibilities in practice settings, (4) social workers' ethical responsibilities as professionals, (5) social workers' ethical responsibilities to the social work profession, and (6) social workers' ethical responsibilities to the broader society.

Some of the standards that follow are enforceable guidelines for professional conduct, and some are aspirational. The extent to which each standard is enforceable is a matter of professional judgment to be exercised by those responsible for reviewing alleged violations of ethical standards.

1. Social Workers' Ethical Responsibilities to Clients

1.01 Commitment to Clients

Social workers' primary responsibility is to promote the well-being of clients. In general, clients' interests are primary. However, social workers' responsibility to the larger society or specific legal obligations may on limited occasions supersede the loyalty owed clients, and clients should be so advised. (Examples include when a social worker is required by law to report that a client has abused a child or has threatened to harm self or others.)

1.02 Self-Determination

Social workers respect and promote the right of clients to self-determination and assist clients in their efforts to identify and clarify their goals. Social workers may limit clients' right to self-determination when, in the social workers' professional judgment, clients' actions or potential actions pose a serious, foreseeable, and imminent risk to themselves or others.

1.03 Informed Consent

(a) Social workers should provide services to clients only in the context of a professional relationship based, when appropriate, on valid informed consent. Social workers should use clear and understandable language to inform clients of the purpose of the services, risks related to the services, limits to services because of the requirements of a third-party payer, relevant costs, reasonable alternatives, clients' right to refuse or withdraw consent, and the time frame covered by the consent. Social workers should provide clients with an opportunity to ask questions.

(b) In instances when clients are not literate or have difficulty understanding the primary language used in the practice setting, social workers should take steps to ensure clients' comprehension. This may include providing clients with a detailed verbal explanation or arranging for a qualified interpreter or translator whenever possible.

(c) In instances when clients lack the capacity to provide informed consent, social workers should protect clients' interests by seeking permission from an appropriate third party, informing clients consistent with the clients' level of understanding. In such instances social workers should seek to ensure that the third party acts in a manner consistent with clients' wishes and interests. Social workers should take reasonable steps to enhance such clients' ability to give informed consent.

(d) In instances when clients are receiving services involuntarily, social workers should provide information about the nature and extent of services and about the extent of clients' right to refuse service.

(e) Social workers who provide services via electronic media (such as computer, telephone, radio, and television) should inform recipients of the limitations and risks associated with such services.

(f) Social workers should obtain clients' informed consent before audiotaping or videotaping clients or permitting observation of services to clients by a third party.

1.04 Competence

(a) Social workers should provide services and represent themselves as competent only within the boundaries of their education, training, license, certification, consultation received, supervised experience, or other relevant professional experience.

(b) Social workers should provide services in substantive areas or use intervention techniques or approaches that are new to them only after engaging in appropriate study, training, consultation, and supervision from people who are competent in those interventions or techniques.

(c) When generally recognized standards do not exist with respect to an emerging area of practice, social workers should exercise careful judgment and take responsible steps (including appropriate education, research, training, consultation, and supervision) to ensure the competence of their work and to protect clients from harm.

1.05 Cultural Competence and Social Diversity

(a) Social workers should understand culture and its function in human behavior and society, recognizing the strengths that exist in all cultures.

(b) Social workers should have a knowledge base of their clients' cultures and be able to demonstrate competence in the provision of services that are sensitive to clients' cultures and to differences among people and cultural groups.

(c) Social workers should obtain education about and seek to understand the nature of social diversity and oppression with respect to race, ethnicity, national origin, color, sex, sexual orientation, age, marital status, political belief, religion, and mental or physical disability.

1.06 Conflicts of Interest

(a) Social workers should be alert to and avoid conflicts of interest that interfere with the exercise of professional discretion and impartial judgment. Social workers should inform clients when a real or potential conflict of interest arises and take reasonable steps to resolve the issue in a manner that makes the clients' interests primary and protects clients' interests to the greatest extent possible. In some cases, protecting clients' interests may require termination of the professional relationship with proper referral of the client.

(b) Social workers should not take unfair advantage of any professional relationship or exploit others to further their personal, religious, political, or business interests.

(c) Social workers should not engage in dual or multiple relationships with clients or former clients in which there is a risk of exploitation or potential harm to the client. In instances when dual or multiple relationships are unavoidable, social workers should take steps to protect clients and are responsible for setting clear, appropriate, and culturally sensitive boundaries. (Dual or multiple relationships occur when social workers relate to clients in more than one relationship, whether professional, social, or business. Dual or multiple relationships can occur simultaneously or consecutively.)

(d) When social workers provide services to two or more people who have a relationship with each other (for example, couples, family members), social workers should clarify with all parties which individuals will be considered clients and the nature of social workers' professional obligations to the various individuals who are receiving services. Social workers who anticipate a conflict of interest among the individuals receiving services or who anticipate having to perform in potentially conflicting roles (for example, when a social worker is asked to testify in a child custody dispute or divorce proceedings involving clients) should clarify their role with the parties involved and take appropriate action to minimize any conflict of interest.

1.07 Privacy and Confidentiality

(a) Social workers should respect clients' right to privacy. Social workers should not solicit private information from clients unless it is essential to providing services or conducting social work evaluation or research. Once private information is shared, standards of confidentiality apply.

(b) Social workers may disclose confidential information when appropriate with valid consent from a client or a person legally authorized to consent on behalf of a client.

(c) Social workers should protect the confidentiality of all information obtained in the course of professional service, except for compelling professional reasons. The general expectation that social workers will keep information confidential does not apply when disclosure is necessary to prevent serious, foreseeable, and imminent harm to a client or other identifiable person. In all instances, social workers should disclose the least amount of confidential information necessary to achieve the desired purpose; only information that is directly relevant to the purpose for which the disclosure is made should be revealed.

(d) Social workers should inform clients, to the extent possible, about the disclosure of confidential information and the potential consequences, when feasible before the disclosure is made. This applies whether social workers disclose confidential information on the basis of a legal requirement or client consent.

(e) Social workers should discuss with clients and other interested parties the nature of confidentiality and limitations of clients' right to confidentiality. Social workers should review with clients circumstances where confidential information may be requested and where disclosure of confidential information may be legally required. This discussion should occur as soon as possible in the social worker-client relationship and as needed throughout the course of the relationship.

(f) When social workers provide counseling services to families, couples, or groups, social workers should seek agreement among the parties involved concerning each individual's right to confidentiality and obligation to preserve the confidentiality of information shared by others. Social workers should inform participants in family, couples, or group counseling that social workers cannot guarantee that all participants will honor such agreements.

(g) Social workers should inform clients involved in family, couples, marital, or group counseling of the social worker's, employer's, and agency's policy concerning the social worker's disclosure of confidential information among the parties involved in the counseling.

(h) Social workers should not disclose confidential information to third-party payers unless clients have authorized such disclosure.

(i) Social workers should not discuss confidential information in any setting unless privacy can be ensured. Social workers should not discuss confidential information in public or semipublic areas such as hallways, waiting rooms, elevators, and restaurants.

(j) Social workers should protect the confidentiality of clients during legal proceedings to the extent permitted by law. When a court of law or other legally authorized body orders social workers to disclose confidential or privileged information without a client's consent and such disclosure could cause harm to the client, social workers should request that the court withdraw the order or limit the order as narrowly as possible or maintain the records under seal, unavailable for public inspection.

(k) Social workers should protect the confidentiality of clients when responding to requests from members of the media.

(l) Social workers should protect the confidentiality of clients' written and electronic records and other sensitive information. Social workers should take reasonable steps to ensure that clients' records are stored in a secure location and that clients' records are not available to others who are not authorized to have access.

(m) Social workers should take precautions to ensure and maintain the confidentiality of information transmitted to other parties through the use of computers, electronic mail, facsimile machines, telephones and telephone answering machines, and other electronic or computer technology. Disclosure of identifying information should be avoided whenever possible.

(n) Social workers should transfer or dispose of clients' records in a manner that protects clients' confidentiality and is consistent with state statutes governing records and social work licensure.

(o) Social workers should take reasonable precautions to protect client confidentiality in the event of the social worker's termination of practice, incapacitation, or death.

(p) Social workers should not disclose identifying information when discussing clients for teaching or training purposes unless the client has consented to disclosure of confidential information.

(q) Social workers should not disclose identifying information when discussing clients with consultants unless the client has consented to disclosure of confidential information or there is a compelling need for such disclosure.

(r) Social workers should protect the confidentiality of deceased clients consistent with the preceding standards.

1.08 Access to Records

(a) Social workers should provide clients with reasonable access to records concerning the clients. Social workers who are concerned that clients' access to their records could cause serious misunderstanding or harm to the client should provide assistance in interpreting the records and consultation with the client regarding the records. Social workers should limit clients' access to their records, or portions of their records, only in exceptional circumstances when there is compelling evidence that such access would cause serious harm to the client. Both clients' requests and the rationale for withholding some or all of the record should be documented in clients' files.

(b) When providing clients with access to their records, social workers should take steps to protect the confidentiality of other individuals identified or discussed in such records.

1.09 Sexual Relationships

(a) Social workers should under no circumstances engage in sexual activities or sexual contact with current clients, whether such contact is consensual or forced.

(b) Social workers should not engage in sexual activities or sexual contact with clients' relatives or other individuals with whom clients maintain a close personal relationship when there is a risk of exploitation or potential harm to the client. Sexual activity or sexual contact with clients' relatives or other individuals with whom clients maintain a personal relationship has the potential to be harmful to the client and may make it difficult for the social worker and client to maintain appropriate professional boundaries. Social workers—not their clients, their clients' relatives, or other individuals with whom the client maintains a personal relationship—assume the full burden for setting clear, appropriate, and culturally sensitive boundaries.

(c) Social workers should not engage in sexual activities or sexual contact with former clients because of the potential for harm to the client. If social workers engage in conduct contrary to this prohibition or claim that an exception to this prohibition is warranted because of extraordinary circumstances, it is social workers—not their clients—who assume the full burden of demonstrating that the former client has not been exploited, coerced, or manipulated, intentionally or unintentionally.

(d) Social workers should not provide clinical services to individuals with whom they have had a prior sexual relationship. Providing clinical services to a former sexual partner has the potential to be harmful to the individual and is likely to make it difficult for the social worker and individual to maintain appropriate professional boundaries.

1.10 Physical Contact

Social workers should not engage in physical contact with clients when there is a possibility of psychological harm to the client as a result of the contact (such as cradling or caressing clients). Social workers who engage in appropriate physical contact with clients are responsible for setting clear, appropriate, and culturally sensitive boundaries that govern such physical contact.

1.11 Sexual Harassment

Social workers should not sexually harass clients. Sexual harassment includes sexual advances, sexual solicitation, requests for sexual favors, and other verbal or physical conduct of a sexual nature.

1.12 Derogatory Language

Social workers should not use derogatory language in their written or verbal communications to or about clients. Social workers should use accurate and respectful language in all communications to and about clients.

1.13 Payment for Services

(a) When setting fees, social workers should ensure that the fees are fair, reasonable, and commensurate with the services performed. Consideration should be given to clients' ability to pay.

(b) Social workers should avoid accepting goods or services from clients as payment for professional services. Bartering arrangements, particularly involving services, create the potential for conflicts of interest, exploitation, and inappropriate boundaries in social workers' relationships with clients. Social workers should explore and may participate in bartering only in very limited circumstances when it can be demonstrated that such arrangements are an accepted practice among professionals in the local community, considered to be essential for the provision of services, negotiated without coercion, and entered into at the client's initiative and with the client's informed consent. Social workers who accept goods or services from clients as payment for professional services assume the full burden of demonstrating that this arrangement will not be detrimental to the client or the professional relationship.

(c) Social workers should not solicit a private fee or other remuneration for providing services to clients who are entitled to such available services through the social workers' employer or agency.

1.14 Clients Who Lack Decision-Making Capacity

When social workers act on behalf of clients who lack the capacity to make informed decisions, social workers should take reasonable steps to safeguard the interests and rights of those clients.

1.15 Interruption of Services

Social workers should make reasonable efforts to ensure continuity of services in the event that services are interrupted by factors such as unavailability, relocation, illness, disability, or death.

1.16 Termination of Services

(a) Social workers should terminate services to clients and professional relationships with them when such services and relationships are no longer required or no longer serve the clients' needs or interests.

(b) Social workers should take reasonable steps to avoid abandoning clients who are still in need of services. Social workers should withdraw services precipitously only under unusual circumstances, giving careful consideration to all factors in the situation and taking care to minimize possible adverse effects. Social workers should assist in making appropriate arrangements for continuation of services when necessary.

(c) Social workers in fee-for-service settings may terminate services to clients who are not paying an overdue balance if the financial contractual arrangements have been made clear to the client, if the client does not pose an imminent danger to self or others, and if the clinical and other consequences of the current nonpayment have been addressed and discussed with the client.

(d) Social workers should not terminate services to pursue a social, financial, or sexual relationship with a client.

(e) Social workers who anticipate the termination or interruption of services to clients should notify clients promptly and seek the transfer, referral, or continuation of services in relation to the clients' needs and preferences.

(f) Social workers who are leaving an employment setting should inform clients of appropriate options for the continuation of services and of the benefits and risks of the options.

2. Social Workers' Ethical Responsibilities to Colleagues

2.01 Respect

(a) Social workers should treat colleagues with respect and should represent accurately and fairly the qualifications, views, and obligations of colleagues.

(b) Social workers should avoid unwarranted negative criticism of colleagues in communications with clients or with other professionals. Unwarranted negative criticism may include demeaning comments that refer to colleagues' level of competence or to individuals' attributes such as race, ethnicity, national origin, color, sex, sexual orientation, age, marital status, political belief, religion, and mental or physical disability.

(c) Social workers should cooperate with social work colleagues and with colleagues of other professions when such cooperation serves the well-being of clients.

2.02 Confidentiality

Social workers should respect confidential information shared by colleagues in the course of their professional relationships and transactions. Social workers should ensure that such colleagues understand social workers' obligation to respect confidentiality and any exceptions related to it.

2.03 Interdisciplinary Collaboration

(a) Social workers who are members of an interdisciplinary team should participate in and contribute to decisions that affect the well-being of clients by drawing on the perspectives, values, and experiences of the social work profession. Professional and ethical obligations of the interdisciplinary team as a whole and of its individual members should be clearly established.

(b) Social workers for whom a team decision raises ethical concerns should attempt to resolve the disagreement through appropriate channels. If the disagreement cannot be resolved, social workers should pursue other avenues to address their concerns consistent with client well-being.

2.04 Disputes Involving Colleagues

(a) Social workers should not take advantage of a dispute between a colleague and an employer to obtain a position or otherwise advance the social workers' own interests.

(b) Social workers should not exploit clients in disputes with colleagues or engage clients in any inappropriate discussion of conflicts between social workers and their colleagues.

2.05 Consultation

(a) Social workers should seek the advice and counsel of colleagues whenever such consultation is in the best interests of clients.

(b) Social workers should keep themselves informed about colleagues' areas of expertise and competencies. Social workers should seek consultation only from colleagues who have demonstrated knowledge, expertise, and competence related to the subject of the consultation.

(c) When consulting with colleagues about clients, social workers should disclose the least amount of information necessary to achieve the purposes of the consultation.

2.06 Referral for Services

(a) Social workers should refer clients to other professionals when the other professionals' specialized knowledge or expertise is needed to serve clients fully or when social workers believe that they are not being effective or making reasonable progress with clients and that additional service is required.

(b) Social workers who refer clients to other professionals should take appropriate steps to facilitate an orderly transfer of responsibility. Social workers who refer clients to other professionals should disclose, with clients' consent, all pertinent information to the new service providers.

(c) Social workers are prohibited from giving or receiving payment for a referral when no professional service is provided by the referring social worker.

2.07 Sexual Relationships

(a) Social workers who function as supervisors or educators should not engage in sexual activities or contact with supervisees, students, trainees, or other colleagues over whom they exercise professional authority.

(b) Social workers should avoid engaging in sexual relationships with colleagues when there is potential for a conflict of interest. Social workers who become involved in, or anticipate becoming involved in, a sexual relationship with a colleague have a duty to transfer professional responsibilities, when necessary, to avoid a conflict of interest.

2.08 Sexual Harassment

Social workers should not sexually harass supervisees, students, trainees, or colleagues. Sexual harassment includes sexual advances, sexual solicitation, requests for sexual favors, and other verbal or physical conduct of a sexual nature.

2.09 Impairment of Colleagues

(a) Social workers who have direct knowledge of a social work colleague's impairment that is due to personal problems, psychosocial distress, substance abuse, or mental health difficulties and that interferes with practice effectiveness should consult with that colleague when feasible and assist the colleague in taking remedial action.

(b) Social workers who believe that a social work colleague's impairment interferes with practice effectiveness and that the colleague has not taken adequate steps to address the impairment should take action through appropriate channels established by employers, agencies, NASW, licensing and regulatory bodies, and other professional organizations.

2.10 Incompetence of Colleagues

(a) Social workers who have direct knowledge of a social work colleague's incompetence should consult with that colleague when feasible and assist the colleague in taking remedial action.

(b) Social workers who believe that a social work colleague is incompetent and has not taken adequate steps to address the incompetence should take action through appropriate channels established by employers, agencies, NASW, licensing and regulatory bodies, and other professional organizations.

2.11 Unethical Conduct of Colleagues

(a) Social workers should take adequate measures to discourage, prevent, expose, and correct the unethical conduct of colleagues.

(b) Social workers should be knowledgeable about established policies and procedures for handling concerns about colleagues' unethical behavior. Social workers should be familiar with national, state, and local procedures for handling ethics complaints. These include policies and procedures created by NASW, licensing and regulatory bodies, employers, agencies, and other professional organizations.

(c) Social workers who believe that a colleague has acted unethically should seek resolution by discussing their concerns with the colleague when feasible and when such discussion is likely to be productive.

(d) When necessary, social workers who believe that a colleague has acted unethically should take action through appropriate formal channels (such as contacting a state licensing board or regulatory body, an NASW committee on inquiry, or other professional ethics committees).

(e) Social workers should defend and assist colleagues who are unjustly charged with unethical conduct.

3. Social Workers' Ethical Responsibilities in Practice Settings

3.01 Supervision and Consultation

(a) Social workers who provide supervision or consultation should have the necessary knowledge and skill to supervise or consult appropriately and should do so only within their areas of knowledge and competence.

(b) Social workers who provide supervision or consultation are responsible for setting clear, appropriate, and culturally sensitive boundaries.

(c) Social workers should not engage in any dual or multiple relationships with supervisees in which there is a risk of exploitation of or potential harm to the supervisee.

(d) Social workers who provide supervision should evaluate supervisees' performance in a manner that is fair and respectful.

3.02 Education and Training

(a) Social workers who function as educators, field instructors for students, or trainers should provide instruction only within their areas of knowledge and competence and should provide instruction based on the most current information and knowledge available in the profession.
(b) Social workers who function as educators or field instructors for students should evaluate students' performance in a manner that is fair and respectful.
(c) Social workers who function as educators or field instructors for students should take reasonable steps to ensure that clients are routinely informed when services are being provided by students.
(d) Social workers who function as educators or field instructors for students should not engage in any dual or multiple relationships with students in which there is a risk of exploitation or potential harm to the student. Social work educators and field instructors are responsible for setting clear, appropriate, and culturally sensitive boundaries.

3.03 Performance Evaluation

Social workers who have responsibility for evaluating the performance of others should fulfill such responsibility in a fair and considerate manner and on the basis of clearly stated criteria.

3.04 Client Records

(a) Social workers should take reasonable steps to ensure that documentation in records is accurate and reflects the services provided.
(b) Social workers should include sufficient and timely documentation in records to facilitate the delivery of services and to ensure continuity of services provided to clients in the future.
(c) Social workers' documentation should protect clients' privacy to the extent that is possible and appropriate and

should include only information that is directly relevant to the delivery of services.

(d) Social workers should store records following the termination of services to ensure reasonable future access. Records should be maintained for the number of years required by state statutes or relevant contracts.

3.05 Billing

Social workers should establish and maintain billing practices that accurately reflect the nature and extent of services provided and that identify who provided the service in the practice setting.

3.06 Client Transfer

(a) When an individual who is receiving services from another agency or colleague contacts a social worker for services, the social worker should carefully consider the client's needs before agreeing to provide services. To minimize possible confusion and conflict, social workers should discuss with potential clients the nature of the clients' current relationship with other service providers and the implications, including possible benefits or risks, of entering into a relationship with a new service provider.

(b) If a new client has been served by another agency or colleague, social workers should discuss with the client whether consultation with the previous service provider is in the client's best interest.

3.07 Administration

(a) Social work administrators should advocate within and outside their agencies for adequate resources to meet clients' needs.

(b) Social workers should advocate for resource allocation procedures that are open and fair. When not all clients' needs can be met, an allocation procedure should be developed that is nondiscriminatory and based on appropriate and consistently applied principles.

(c) Social workers who are administrators should take reasonable steps to ensure that adequate agency or organizational resources are available to provide appropriate staff supervision. .

(d) Social work administrators should take reasonable steps to ensure that the working environment for which they are responsible is consistent with and encourages compliance with the *NASW Code of Ethics*. Social work administrators should take reasonable steps to eliminate any conditions in their organizations that violate, interfere with, or discourage compliance with the *Code*.

3.08   Continuing Education and Staff Development

Social work administrators and supervisors should take reasonable steps to provide or arrange for continuing education and staff development for all staff for whom they are responsible. Continuing education and staff development should address current knowledge and emerging developments related to social work practice and ethics.

3.09   Commitments to Employers

(a) Social workers generally should adhere to commitments made to employers and employing organizations.

(b) Social workers should work to improve employing agencies' policies and procedures and the efficiency and effectiveness of their services.

(c) Social workers should take reasonable steps to ensure that employers are aware of social workers' ethical obligations as set forth in the *NASW Code of Ethics* and of the implications of those obligations for social work practice.

(d) Social workers should not allow an employing organization's policies, procedures, regulations, or administrative orders to interfere with their ethical practice of social work. Social workers should take reasonable steps to ensure that their employing organizations' practices are consistent with the *NASW Code of Ethics*.

(e) Social workers should act to prevent and eliminate discrimination in the employing organization's work assignments and in its employment policies and practices.

(f) Social workers should accept employment or arrange student field placements only in organizations that exercise fair personnel practices.

(g) Social workers should be diligent stewards of the resources of their employing organizations, wisely conserving funds where appropriate and never misappropriating funds or using them for unintended purposes.

3.10 Labor-Management Disputes

(a) Social workers may engage in organized action, including the formation of and participation in labor unions, to improve services to clients and working conditions.

(b) The actions of social workers who are involved in labor-management disputes, job actions, or labor strikes should be guided by the profession's values, ethical principles, and ethical standards. Reasonable differences of opinion exist among social workers concerning their primary obligation as professionals during an actual or threatened labor strike or job action. Social workers should carefully examine relevant issues and their possible impact on clients before deciding on a course of action.

4. Social Workers' Ethical Responsibilities as Professionals

4.01 Competence

(a) Social workers should accept responsibility or employment only on the basis of existing competence or the intention to acquire the necessary competence.

(b) Social workers should strive to become and remain proficient in professional practice and the performance of professional functions. Social workers should critically examine and keep current with emerging knowledge relevant to social work. Social workers should routinely review the professional literature and participate in continuing education relevant to social work practice and social work ethics.

(c) Social workers should base practice on recognized knowledge, including empirically based knowledge, relevant to social work and social work ethics.

4.02 Discrimination

Social workers should not practice, condone, facilitate, or collaborate with any form of discrimination on the basis of race, ethnicity, national origin, color, sex, sexual orientation, age, marital status, political belief, religion, or mental or physical disability.

4.03 Private Conduct

Social workers should not permit their private conduct to interfere with their ability to fulfill their professional responsibilities.

4.04 Dishonesty, Fraud, and Deception

Social workers should not participate in, condone, or be associated with dishonesty, fraud, or deception.

4.05 Impairment

(a) Social workers should not allow their own personal problems, psychosocial distress, legal problems, substance abuse, or mental health difficulties to interfere with their professional judgment and performance or to jeopardize the best interests of people for whom they have a professional responsibility.

(b) Social workers whose personal problems, psychosocial distress, legal problems, substance abuse, or mental health difficulties interfere with their professional judgment and performance should immediately seek consultation and take appropriate remedial action by seeking professional help, making adjustments in workload, terminating practice, or taking any other steps necessary to protect clients and others.

4.06 Misrepresentation

(a) Social workers should make clear distinctions between statements made and actions engaged in as a private individual and as a representative of the social work profession, a professional social work organization, or the social worker's employing agency.

(b) Social workers who speak on behalf of professional social work organizations should accurately represent the official and authorized positions of the organizations.

(c) Social workers should ensure that their representations to clients, agencies, and the public of professional qualifications, credentials, education, competence, affiliations, services provided, or results to be achieved are accurate. Social workers should claim only those relevant professional credentials they actually possess and take steps to correct any inaccuracies or misrepresentations of their credentials by others.

4.07 Solicitations

(a) Social workers should not engage in uninvited solicitation of potential clients who, because of their circumstances, are vulnerable to undue influence, manipulation, or coercion.

(b) Social workers should not engage in solicitation of testimonial endorsements (including solicitation of consent to use a client's prior statement as a testimonial endorsement) from current clients or from other people who, because of their particular circumstances, are vulnerable to undue influence.

4.08 Acknowledging Credit

(a) Social workers should take responsibility and credit, including authorship credit, only for work they have actually performed and to which they have contributed.

(b) Social workers should honestly acknowledge the work of and the contributions made by others.

5. Social Workers' Ethical Responsibilities to the Social Work Profession

5.01 Integrity of the Profession

(a) Social workers should work toward the maintenance and promotion of high standards of practice.

(b) Social workers should uphold and advance the values, ethics, knowledge, and mission of the profession. Social workers should protect, enhance, and improve the integrity of the profession through appropriate study and research, active discussion, and responsible criticism of the profession.

(c) Social workers should contribute time and professional expertise to activities that promote respect for the value, integrity, and competence of the social work profession. These activities may include teaching, research, consultation, service, legislative testimony, presentations in the community, and participation in their professional organizations.

(d) Social workers should contribute to the knowledge base of social work and share with colleagues their knowledge related to practice, research, and ethics. Social workers should seek to contribute to the profession's literature and to share their knowledge at professional meetings and conferences.

(e) Social workers should act to prevent the unauthorized and unqualified practice of social work.

5.02 Evaluation and Research

(a) Social workers should monitor and evaluate policies, the implementation of programs, and practice interventions.

(b) Social workers should promote and facilitate evaluation and research to contribute to the development of knowledge.

(c) Social workers should critically examine and keep current with emerging knowledge relevant to social work and fully use evaluation and research evidence in their professional practice.

(d) Social workers engaged in evaluation or research should carefully consider possible consequences and should follow guidelines developed for the protection of evaluation and research participants. Appropriate institutional review boards should be consulted.

(e) Social workers engaged in evaluation or research should obtain voluntary and written informed consent from participants, when appropriate, without any implied or actual deprivation or penalty for refusal to participate; without undue inducement to participate; and with due regard for participants' well-being, privacy, and dignity. Informed consent should include information about the nature, extent, and duration of the participation requested and disclosure of the risks and benefits of participation in the research.

(f) When evaluation or research participants are incapable of giving informed consent, social workers should provide an appropriate explanation to the participants, obtain the participants' assent to the extent they are able, and obtain written consent from an appropriate proxy.

(g) Social workers should never design or conduct evaluation or research that does not use consent procedures, such as certain forms of naturalistic observation and archival research, unless rigorous and responsible review of the research has found it to be justified because of its prospective scientific, educational, or applied value and unless equally effective alternative procedures that do not involve waiver of consent are not feasible.

(h) Social workers should inform participants of their right to withdraw from evaluation and research at any time without penalty.

(i) Social workers should take appropriate steps to ensure that participants in evaluation and research have access to appropriate supportive services.

(j) Social workers engaged in evaluation or research should protect participants from unwarranted physical or mental distress, harm, danger, or deprivation.

(k) Social workers engaged in the evaluation of services should discuss collected information only for professional purposes and only with people professionally concerned with this information.

(l) Social workers engaged in evaluation or research should ensure the anonymity or confidentiality of participants and of the data obtained from them. Social workers should inform participants of any limits of confidentiality, the measures that will be taken to ensure confidentiality, and when any records containing research data will be destroyed.

(m) Social workers who report evaluation and research results should protect participants' confidentiality by omitting identifying information unless proper consent has been obtained authorizing disclosure.

(n) Social workers should report evaluation and research findings accurately. They should not fabricate or falsify results and should take steps to correct any errors later found in published data using standard publication methods.

(o) Social workers engaged in evaluation or research should be alert to and avoid conflicts of interest and dual relationships with participants, should inform participants when a real or potential conflict of interest arises, and should take steps to resolve the issue in a manner that makes participants' interests primary.

(p) Social workers should educate themselves, their students, and their colleagues about responsible research practices.

6. Social Workers' Ethical Responsibilities to the Broader Society

6.01 Social Welfare

Social workers should promote the general welfare of society, from local to global levels, and the development of people, their communities, and their environments. Social workers should advocate for living conditions conducive to the fulfillment of basic human needs and should promote social, economic, political, and cultural values and institutions that are compatible with the realization of social justice.

6.02 Public Participation

Social workers should facilitate informed participation by the public in shaping social policies and institutions.

6.03 Public Emergencies

Social workers should provide appropriate professional services in public emergencies to the greatest extent possible.

6.04 Social and Political Action

(a) Social workers should engage in social and political action that seeks to ensure that all people have equal access to the resources, employment, services, and opportunities they require to meet their basic human needs and to develop fully. Social workers should be aware of the impact of the political arena on practice and should advocate for changes in policy and legislation to improve social conditions in order to meet basic human needs and promote social justice.

(b) Social workers should act to expand choice and opportunity for all people, with special regard for vulnerable, disadvantaged, oppressed, and exploited people and groups.

(c) Social workers should promote conditions that encourage respect for cultural and social diversity within the United States and globally. Social workers should promote policies and practices that demonstrate respect for difference, support the expansion of cultural knowledge and resources, advocate for programs and institutions that demonstrate cultural competence, and promote policies that safeguard the rights of and confirm equity and social justice for all people.

(d) Social workers should act to prevent and eliminate domination of, exploitation of, and discrimination against any person, group, or class on the basis of race, ethnicity, national origin, color, sex, sexual orientation, age, marital status, political belief, religion, or mental or physical disability.

Appendix F

AN ILLUSTRATIVE
INFORMED CONSENT STATEMENT
USED IN AN OUTPATIENT PRACTICE

Patient Information/Informed Consent
Dr. _____

This provides some basic information about psychological treatment. Please read and sign below to indicate that you have reviewed this information.

LENGTH OF TREATMENT

Psychotherapy often involves regular weekly sessions that are up to 50 minutes long. Many problems can be resolved in 6 to 10 visits, but the number needed depends greatly on the nature of the problem and your individual situation.

CONFIDENTIALITY

Psychologists have both a legal and a professional obligation to protect your privacy and maintain your confidentiality. However, there are several limitations to confidentiality that you should be aware of: Insurance carriers and HMOs will typically require that the diagnosis be communicated to them; in many cases information establishing the need for treatment will be required, as well. Other limitations to confidentiality include, but are not limited to, court orders, situations in which life (yours, a child's, or another's) is in danger, and supervisory consultations for therapists in training. Records are released only with your written permission. If a clinic physician referred you, your therapist may also communicate your diagnosis and treatment progress to that doctor unless you direct otherwise.

EMERGENCIES

When your therapist is unavailable, arrangements can be made for coverage or telephone contact as necessary. The hospital operator (# here) can page your therapist in most cases.

PHYSICIAN CONTACT

Physical and psychological symptoms often interact, and we encourage you to seek medical consultation as needed. In addition, medication may sometimes be helpful for psychological disorders. When appropriate, consultation with your primary care physician or referral for psychiatric consultation will be offered.

FREEDOM TO WITHDRAW

You have the right to end therapy at any time and are obligated only to pay for completed sessions. If you wish, your therapist can provide you with names of other qualified psychotherapists.

FEE POLICIES

Our billing rates and fee policies are explained on a separate sheet. Although we will assist with the billing and insurance reimbursement problems, please be aware that charges for services are the patient's responsibility.

INFORMED CONSENT

I have read and understood the preceding statement, have had the opportunity to ask questions about it, and agree to begin treatment.

Name: _____ Date: _____

Witnessed by (Therapist): _____

REFERENCES

Abraham v. Zaslow, Docket No. 245862 (Sup. Ct. Santa Clara County, Oct. 26, 1970). Reported in Glenn R. (1974).

American Association for Marriage and Family Therapy. (2001). *Code of Ethics.* Washington, DC: Author.

American Association of State Psychology Boards. (1985). *Guidelines for Computer Based Assessment and Interpretation.* New York: Author.

American Counseling Association. (1995) *Code of Ethics and Standards of Practice.* Alexandria, VA: Author.

American Educational Research Association, American Psychological Association, & National Council on Measurement in Education. (1999). *Standards for Educational and Psychological Testing.* Washington, DC: American Psychological Association.

American Psychiatric Association. (1997). What makes good practice guidelines? *Psychiatric News,* January 17, 1997. Retrieved April 14, 2001, from http://www.psych.org/pnews/97-01-17/good.html

American Psychiatric Association. (2000). *Diagnostic and Statistical Manual for Mental Disorders (DSM-IV-TR;* 4th ed. text rev.). Washington, DC: Author.

American Psychiatric Association. (2001). *The Principles of Medical Ethics With Annotations Especially Applicable to Psychiatry.* Washington, DC: Author.

American Psychological Association. (1986). *Guidelines for Computer Based Tests and Interpretations.* Washington, DC: Author.

American Psychological Association. (1987). General guidelines for providers of psychological services. *American Psychologist, 42,* 712-723.

American Psychological Association. (1993). Record keeping guide-lines. *American Psychologist, 48,* 984-986.

American Psychological Association. (2002). Ethical Principles of Psychologists and Code of Conduct. *American Psychologist, 57,* 1060-1073.

Appelbaum, P. S. (1985). Tarasoff and the clinician: Problems in fulfilling the duty to protect. *American Journal of Psychiatry, 142,* 425-429.

Appelbaum, P. S. (1990). The parable of the forensic psychiatrist: Ethics and the problem of doing harm. *International Journal of Law and Psychiatry, 13*(4), 249-259.

Appelbaum, P. S. (1993). Legal liability and managed care. *American Psychologist, 48,* 251-257.

Ascher, L. M., & Turner, R. M. (1980). A comparison of two methods for the administration of paradoxical intention. *Behavior Research and Treatment, 18,* 121-126.

Barak, A. (1999). Psychological applications on the Internet: A discipline on the threshold of a new millennium. *Applied and Preventive Psychology, 8,* 231-246.

Beauchamp, T. L., & Childress, J. F. (2001). *Principles of Biomedical Ethics* (5th ed.). New York: Oxford University Press.

Beck, J. (1982). When the patient threatens violence: An empirical study of clinical practice after Tarasoff. *Bulletin of the American Academy of Psychiatry and Law, 10,* 189-201.

Beier, E. G., & Young, D. (1984). *The Silent Language of Psychotherapy* (2nd ed.). Chicago: Aldine Publishing.

Bennett, B. E., Bryant, B. K., VandenBos, G. R., & Greenwood, A. (1990). *Professional Liability and Risk Management.* Washington, DC: American Psychological Association.

Bentham, J. (1948). *An Introduction to the Principles of Morals and Legislation.* New York: Hafar Publishing. (Original work published 1863)

Bergeron, L. R., & Gray, B. (2003, January). Ethical dilemmas of reporting suspected elder abuse. *Social Work, 48*(1), 96-105.

Berman, A. L., & Cohen-Sandler, R. (1983). Suicide and malpractice: Expert testimony and the standard of care. *Professional Psychology: Research and Practice, 14,* 6-19.

Berndt, D. J. (1983). Ethical and professional considerations in psychological assessment. *Professional Psychology: Research and Practice, 14,* 580-587.

Bernstein, B. L., & LeComte, C. (1981). Licensure and psychology: Alternative directions. *Professional Psychology, 12,* 200-208.

Bersoff, D. (1976). Psychologists as protectors and policemen: New roles as a result of Tarasoff? *Professional Psychology, 7,* 267-273.

Bongar, B. (1991). *The Suicidal Patient: Clinical and Legal Standards of Care.* Washington, DC: American Psychological Association.

Bouhoutsos, J., Holroyd, J., Lerman, H., Forer, B. R., & Greenberg, M. (1983). Sexual intimacy between psychotherapists and patients. *Professional Psychology: Research and Practice, 14,* 185-196.

Brodsky, S. L. (1991). *Testifying in Court: Guidelines and Maxims for the Expert Witness.* Washington, DC: American Psychological Association.

Budman, S. H. (2000). Behavioral health care dot-com and beyond: Computer-mediated communications in mental health and substance abuse treatment. *American Psychologist, 55*(11), 1290-1300.

Butz, R. A. (1985). Reporting child abuse and confidentiality in counseling: Implications for social work. *Social Casework, 66,* 83-90.

Campbell, D. T., & Stanley, J. C. (1963). *Experimental and Quasi-Experimental Designs for Research.* Chicago: Rand McNally.

Candee, D. (1985). Classical ethics and live patient simulations in the moral education of health care professionals. In M. W. Berkowitz & F. Oser (Eds.), *Moral Education: Theory and Application* (pp. 297-318). Hillsdale, NJ: Lawrence Erlbaum.

Caplan, A. (1982). On privacy and confidentiality in social science research. In T. R. Beauchamp, R. R. Faden, R. J. Wallace, & L. Walters (Eds.), *Ethical Issues in Social Science Research* (pp. 315-325). Baltimore, MD: Johns Hopkins.

Caruth, E. G. (1985). Secret bearer or secret barer. *Contemporary Psychoanalysis, 4,* 548-562.

Cohen, R. J. (1979). *Malpractice: A Guide for Mental Health Professionals.* New York: The Free Press.

Cohen, R. J., & Mariano, W. E. (1982). *Legal Guidebook in Mental Health.* New York: The Free Press.

Committee on Professional Practice and Standards. (2003, December). Legal issues in the professional practice of psychology. *Professional Psychology: Research and Practice, 34*(6), 595-600.

Corey, G., Corey, M. S., & Callanan, P. (1988). *Issues and Ethics in the Helping Professions* (3rd ed.). Monterey, CA: Brooks/Cole.

Crenshaw, W. B., & Lichtenberg, J. W. (1993, Spring). Child abuse and the limits of confidentiality: Forewarning practices. *Behavioral Sciences and the Law, 11*(2), 181-192.

Davidson, J. R., & Davidson, T. (1996, August). Confidentiality and managed care: Ethical and legal concerns. *Health and Social Work, 21*(3), 208-215.

Dawson, C. S. (1981). *Truthtelling, Paternalism, and Autonomy in Psychotherapy.* Unpublished doctoral dissertation, California School of Professional Psychology, Berkeley, CA.

DeKraii, M. B., & Sales, B. D. (1984). Confidential communications of psychotherapists. *Psychotherapy, 21,* 293-318.

Dimatteo, R. M., & Hendricks, S. F. (1982). *Interpersonal Issues in Health Care.* New York: Academic Press.

Division of Psychology and Law. (1991). *Guidelines for the Practice of Forensic Psychology.* Washington, DC: Author.

Drew, J., Stoeckle, J. D., & Billings, J. A. (1983). Tips, status, and sacrifice: Gift giving in the doctor-patient relationship. *Social Science and Medicine, 17,* 399-404.

Dubin, S. S. (1972). Obsolescence or life-long education: A choice for the professional. *American Psychologist, 27,* 486-496.

Ende, J. (1983, August 12). Feedback in clinical medical education. *Journal of the American Medical Association, 250*(6), 777-781.

Erickson, S. H. (1990). Counseling irresponsible AIDS patients: Guidelines for decision making. *Journal of Counseling and Development, 68*(4), 454-455.

Ethics Committee of the American Psychological Association. (1988). Trends in ethics cases, common pitfalls, and published resources. *American Psychologist, 43,* 564-572.

Faden, R. R., Beauchamp, T. L., & King, N. M. (1986). *A History and Theory of Informed Consent.* New York: Oxford University Press.

Faust, D. (1986). Research on human judgment and its application to clinical practice. *Professional Psychology: Research and Practice, 17,* 420-430.

Faustman, W. (1982). Legal and ethical issues in debt collection strategies of professional psychologists. *Professional Psychology: Research and Practice, 13,* 208-214.

Felthous, A. (1989). The ever-confusing jurisprudence of the psychotherapist's duty to protect. *Journal of Psychiatry & Law, 17*(4), 575-594.

Fisher, C. B., & Fried, A. L. (2003, Spring-Summer). Internet-mediated psychological services and the American Psychological Association Ethics Code. *Psychotherapy: Theory, Research, Practice, and Training, 40*(1-2), 103-111.

Foxhall, K. (2000). How would your practice records look to the FBI? *The APA Monitor, 30*(1), 50-52.

Fretz, B., & Mills, D. (1980). *Licensing and Certification of Psychologists and Counselors.* San Francisco: Jossey-Bass.

Freudenberger, H. (1982). Burnout and stress in mental health providers. In G. VandenBos (Ed.), *Professionals in Distress* (pp. 135-152). Washington, DC: American Psychological Association.

Garb, H. N. (1991). The trained psychologist as expert witness. *Professional Psychology: Research and Practice, 37,* 451-467.

Gaylin, W. (1982). The competence of children: No longer all or none. *Hastings Center Report, 12,* 33-38.

Geraty, R. D., Hendren, R., & Flaa, C. J. (1992). Ethical perspectives on managed care as it relates to child and adolescent psychiatry. *Journal of the American Academy of Child and Adolescent Psychiatry, 31*(3), 398-402.

Gerts, B. (1981). *The Moral Rules.* New York: Ballantine.

Glass, L. L. (2003). The gray areas of boundary crossings and violations. *American Journal of Psychotherapy, 57*(4), 429-444.

Golding, S. L. (1990). Mental health professionals and the courts: The ethics of expertise. *International Journal of Law and Psychiatry, 13*(4), 281-307.

Gomes-Schwartz, B., Hadley, S. W., & Strupp, H. (1978). Individual therapy and behavior therapy. *Annual Review of Psychology, 29,* 435-471.

Goodstein, L. (1983). The correct policy on co-payments. *APA Monitor,* p. 5.

Grams, R. R., & Moyer, E. H. (1997). The search for the elusive electronic medical record system—Medical liability, the missing factor. *Journal of Medical Systems, 21*(1), 1-10.

Grohol, J. M. (1999). Best practices in e-therapy: Confidentiality and privacy. Boston: Author. Retrieved October 24, 2000, from the World Wide Web: http://psychcentral.com/best/best2.htm

Gross, S. J. (1978). The myth of professional licensing. *American Psychologist, 33,* 1009-1016.

Groth-Marnat, G. (1984). *Handbook of Psychological Assessment.* New York: Van Nostrand Reinhold.

Haas, L. J. (1993). Competence and quality in the performance of forensic psychologists. *Ethics and Behavior, 3,* 251-266.

Haas, L. J., Benedict, J. G., & Kobos, J. C. (1996). Psychotherapy by telephone: Risks and benefits for psychologists and consumers. *Professional Psychology: Research and Practice, 27,* 97-102.

Haas, L. J., & Cummings, N. A. (1991). Managed outpatient mental health plans: Clinical, ethical and practical guidelines for participation. *Professional Psychology: Research and Practice, 22,* 45-51.

Haas, L. J., & Hall, J. H. (1990). Impaired or unethical? Issues for colleagues and ethics committees. *The Register Report, 3,* 2-5.

Haas, L. J., Malouf, J. L., & Mayerson, N. H. (1986). Ethical dilemmas in psychological practice: Results of a national survey. *Professional Psychology: Research and Practice, 17,* 316-321.

Hall, J. E., & Hare-Mustin, R. T. (1983). Sanctions and the diversity of ethical complaints against psychologists. *American Psychologist, 38,* 714-729.

Hare-Mustin, R. T., Maracek, J., Kaplan, A., & Liss-Levinson, N. (1979). Rights of clients, responsibilities of therapists. *American Psychologist, 34,* 3-16.

Hathaway, S. R., & McKinley, J. C. (1948). *Minnesota Multiphasic Personality Inventory.* Minneapolis, MN: The Psychological Corporation.

Hathaway, S. R., & McKinley, J. C. (1989). *Minnesota Multiphasic Personality Inventory-2.* Minneapolis, MN: University of Minnesota Press.

Heinlen, K. T., Welfel, E. R., Richmond, E. N., & Rak, C. F. (2003, Winter). The scope of WebCounseling: A survey of services and compliance with NBCC Standards for the ethical practice of WebCounseling. *Journal of Counseling and Development, 81*(1), 61-69.

Helbok, C. M. (2003, October). The practice of psychology in rural communities: Potential ethical dilemmas. *Ethics and Behavior, 13*(4), 367-384.

Hills, H. I., Gruszkos, J. R., & Strong, S. R. (1985). Attribution and the double bind in paradoxical interventions. *Psychotherapy, 22,* 779-785.

Hoffman, I. (1979). Psychological versus medical psychotherapy. *Professional Psychology, 10,* 571-595.

Holder, A. (1985). *Legal Issues in Pediatrics and Adolescent Medicine*. New Haven: Yale University Press.

Hundert, E. M. (1998, July-August). Looking a gift horse in the mouth: The ethics of gift-giving in psychiatry. *Harvard Review of Psychiatry, 6*(2), 114-117.

Hunsley, J. (1988). Conceptions and misconceptions about the context of paradoxical therapy. *Professional Psychology: Research and Practice, 19*, 553-559.

Huprich, S. K., Fuller, K. M., & Schneider, R. B. (2003, July). Divergent ethical perspectives on the duty-to-warn principle with HIV patients. *Ethics and Behavior, 13*(3), 263-278.

Jablonski v. United States, 712 F.2d 391 (9th Cir. 1983).

Jacob, S., & Hartshorne, T. S. (2003). *Ethics and Law for School Psychologists* (4th ed.). Hoboken, NJ: Wiley.

Jaffee v. Redmond, 116 S. Ct. 1923 (1996).

Jennings, F. L. (1992). Ethics of rural practice: Psychological practice in small towns and rural areas [Special issue]. *Psychotherapy in Private Practice, 10*(3), 85-104.

Jonsen, A. R., Siegler, M., & Winslade, W. J. (1998). *Clinical Ethics* (4th ed.). New York: McGraw-Hill.

Kahneman, D., & Tversky, A. (1981). The framing of decisions and the psychology of choice. *Science, 211*, 453-458.

Kahneman, D., & Tversky, A. (1984). Choices, values, and frames. *American Psychologist, 39*, 341-350.

Kalichman, S. C., & Craig. M. E. (1991). Professional psychologists' decisions to report suspected child abuse: Clinical and situational influences. *Professional Psychology, 22*(1), 84-89.

Kane, M. T. (1982). The validity of licensure examinations. *American Psychologist, 37*, 911-918.

Kaufman, M. (1991). Post-Tarasoff legal developments and the mental health literature. *Bulletin of the Menninger Clinic, 55*, 308-322.

Keeton, W. P. (Ed.). (1984). *Prosser and Keeton on the Law of Torts* (5th ed.). St. Paul, MN: West.

Kegeles, S., Catania, J., & Coates, T. (1988). Intentions to communicate positive HIV-antibody status to sex partners [Letter to the editor]. *Journal of the American Medical Association, 259*, 216-217.

Keith-Spiegel, P. (1977). The violation of ethical principles due to ignorance or poor professional judgment versus willful disregard. *Professional Psychology, 8*, 288-296.

Kennedy, P. F., Vandehey, M., Norman, W. B., & Diekhoff, G. (2003, June). Recommendations for risk-management practices. *Professional Psychology: Research and Practice, 34*(3), 309-311.

King, J. H. (1986). *The Law of Medical Malpractice* (2nd ed.). St. Paul, MN: West.

Kinzie, J. D., Holmes, J. L., & Arent, J. (1985). Patients' release of medical records. *Hospital and Community Psychiatry, 36,* 843-847.

Knapp, S., & VandeCreek, L. (1982). Tarasoff: Five years later. *Professional Psychology, 13,* 511-516.

Knapp, S., & VandeCreek, L. (1987). *Privileged Communications in the Mental Health Professions.* New York: Van Nostrand Reinhold.

Knapp, S., & VandeCreek, L. (1990). *What Every Therapist Should Know About AIDS.* Sarasota, FL: Professional Resource Exchange.

Knapp, S., & VandeCreek, L. (2003, June). An overview of the major changes in the 2002 APA Ethics Code. *Professional Psychology: Research and Practice, 34*(3), 301-308.

Koocher, G. P. (2004, August). Ethical and legal issues in professional practice transitions. *Professional Psychology: Research and Practice, 34*(4), 383-387.

Koocher, G. P., & Keith-Spiegel, P. (1998). *Ethics in Psychology: Professional Standards and Cases* (2nd ed.). New York: Oxford University Press.

Laliotis, D. A., & Grayson, J. H. (1985). Psychologist heal thyself: What is available for the impaired psychologist? *American Psychologist, 40,* 84-96.

Lamb, D. H., Catanzaro, S. J., & Moorman, A. S. (2004, June). A preliminary look at how psychologists identify, evaluate, and proceed when faced with possible multiple relationship dilemmas. *Professional Psychology: Research and Practice, 35*(3), 248-254.

Levine, M. L., & Lyon-Levine, M. (1984). Ethical conflicts at the interface of advocacy and psychiatry. *Hospital and Community Psychiatry, 35,* 665-666.

Lowman, R. L. (Ed.). (1991). Introduction to a special section on managed mental health care. Additional info: Managed mental health care. *Professional Psychology: Research and Practice, 22,* 5-59.

Macklin, R. (1991). HIV infected psychiatric patients: Beyond confidentiality. *Ethics and Behavior, 1*(1), 3-20.

Marsh, D. T., & Magee, R. D. (Eds.). (1997). *Ethical and Legal Issues in Professional Practice With Families.* New York: Wiley.

Matarazzo, J. D. (1986). Computerized clinical psychological test interpretations: Unvalidated plus all mean and no sigma. *American Psychologist, 4,* 14-24.

McGee, T. F. (2004, August). Observations on the retirement of professional psychologists. *Professional Psychology: Research and Practice, 34*(4), 388-395.

McGuire, J. M., Toal, P., & Blau, B. (1985). The adult clients perception of confidentiality in the therapeutic relationship. *Professional Psychology: Research and Practice, 16,* 375-384.

Medical Information Bureau. (1993). *Your Rights to Your File.* Boston: Author.

Melton, G. B. (1981). Children's participation in treatment planning: Psychological and legal issues. *Professional Psychology: Research and Practice, 12,* 246-252.

Melton, G. B., Petrila, J., Poythress, N. G., & Slogobin, C. (1997). *Psychological Evaluations for the Courts* (2nd ed.). New York: Guilford.

Mills, D. (1986). Ethics education and adjudication in psychology. *American Psychologist, 39,* 669-675.

Monahan, J. (Ed.). (1980). *Who Is the Client?: The Ethics of Psychological Intervention in the Criminal Justice System.* Washington, DC: American Psychological Association.

Nagy, T. (1987, November). Electronic ethics. *The APA Monitor,* p. 3.

National Association of Social Workers. (1999). *Code of Ethics.* Washington, DC: Author.

Norcross, J. C., & Prochaska, J. O. (1983). Psychotherapist's perspectives on treating themselves and their client for psychic distress. *Professional Psychology: Research and Practice, 14,* 642-655.

Norris, D. M., Gutheil, T. G., & Strasburger, L. H. (2003, April). This couldn't happen to me: Boundary problems and sexual misconduct in the psychotherapy relationship. *Psychiatric Services, 54*(4), 517-522.

Office of Civil Rights. (2003). Medical privacy—National standards to protect the privacy of personal health information. Retrieved on August 30, 2004, from www.hhs.gov/ocr/hipaa/privacy.html

Patel, V. L., & Groen, G. J. (1991). The general and specific nature of medical expertise: A critical look. In K. A. Ericsson & J. Smith

(Eds.), *Toward a General Theory of Expertise: Prospects and Limits* (pp. 93-125). New York: Cambridge University Press.

Peck v. The Counseling Service of Addison County, 499 A. 2d 422 (Vt. 1985).

Pellegrino, E. D. (1979). Toward a reconstruction of medical morality: The primacy of the act of profession and the fact of illness. *The Journal of Medicine and Philosophy, 4,* 32-56.

Petersen v. State, 671 P.2d 230 (Wa. 1983).

Petrila, J. P., & Sadoff, R. L. (1992). Confidentiality and the family as caregiver. *Hospital and Community Psychiatry, 43*(2), 136-139.

P. L. 104-191. (1996). The Health Insurance Portability and Accountability Act (HIPAA) of 1996. *United States Code.* Washington, DC: Government Printing Office.

Plotkin, R. (1981). When rights collide: Parents, children and consent to treatment. *Journal of Pediatric Psychology, 6,* 121-130.

Pope, K. S. (1985, August). *Diagnosis and Treatment of the Therapist-Patient Sex Syndrome.* Paper presented at the annual convention of the American Psychological Association, Los Angeles, CA.

Ragusea, A. S., & VandeCreek, L. (2003, Spring-Summer). Suggestions for the ethical practice of online psychotherapy. *Psychotherapy: Theory, Research, Practice, and Training, 40*(1-2), 94-102.

Reamer, F. G. (2003, January). Boundary issues in social work: Managing dual relationships. *Social Work, 48*(1), 121-133.

Reed, G. M., McGauthlin, J. C., & Miholland, K. (2000). Ten interdisciplinary principles for professional practice in telehealth: Implications for psychology. *Professional Psychology: Research and Practice, 31,* 170-178.

Rest, J. R. (1982). A psychologist looks at the teaching of ethics— Moral development and moral education. *The Hastings Center Report, 12,* 29-36.

Rohrbaugh, T. (1982). Varieties of paradoxical therapy. *Professional Psychology: Research and Practice, 12,* 125-132.

Roy, J., & Freeman, L. (1976). *Betrayal: Based on the Personal Account of Julie Ray.* New York: Stein & Day.

Rubanowitz, D. E. (1987). Public attitudes toward psychotherapist-client confidentiality. *Professional Psychology: Research and Practice, 18,* 613-618.

Ryabik, J. E., Olson, K. R., & Kleim, D. M. (1984). Ethical issues in computerized psychological assessment. *Professional Practice of Psychology, 5,* 31-39.

Schetky, D. H., & Cavanaugh, J. L. (1982). Child psychiatric practice: Psychiatric malpractice. *Journal of the American Academy of Child Psychiatry, 21,* 521-526.

Schwartz, G. (1989). Confidentiality revisited. *Social Work, 34*(3), 223-226.

Schwitzgebel, R. L., & Schwitzgebel, R. K. (1980). *Law and Psychological Practice.* New York: Wiley.

Sell, J. M., Gottlieb, M. C., & Schoenfield, L. (1986). Ethical considerations of social/romantic relationships with present and former clients. *Professional Psychology: Research and Practice, 17,* 504-508.

Shapiro, D. L. (1990). Problems encountered in the preparation and presentation of expert testimony. In E. Margenau (Ed.), *The Encyclopedic Handbook of Private Practice* (pp. 739-758). New York: Gardner.

Shapiro, D. L. (1992). Ethical problems in the suppression of data. *Forensic Reports, 5*(2), 163-168.

Silk, K. R., & Yager, J. (2003, July). Suggested guidelines for E-mail communications in psychiatric practice. *Journal of Clinical Psychiatry, 64*(7), 799-806.

Stockman, A. F. (1990). Dual relationships in rural mental health practice: An ethical dilemma. *Journal of Rural Community Psychology, 11*(2), 31-45.

Stromberg, C. (1992, August). *"Managed Care" How to Practice Ethically.* Paper presented at the annual convention of the American Psychological Association, Washington, DC.

Suisson, E. L., VandeCreek, L., & Knapp, S. (1987). Thorough record keeping: A good defense in a litigious era. *Professional Psychology: Research and Practice, 18,* 498-502.

Swenson, E. (1986). Legal liability for a patient's suicide. *Journal of Psychiatry & Law, 14*(3-4), 409-434.

Szasz, T. (1986). The case against suicide prevention. *American Psychologist, 41,* 806-812.

Tarasoff v. Board of Regents of the University of California, 551 P.2d 334 (Cal. 1976).

Tierney, W. M., Overhage, J. M., Takesue, B. Y., Harris, L. E., Murray, M. D., Vargo, D. L., & McDonald, C. J. (1995). Computerizing guidelines to improve care and patient outcomes: The example of heart failure. *Journal of the American Medical Informatics Association, 2*(5), 316-322.

VandeCreek, L., & Knapp, S. (2001). *Tarasoff and Beyond: Legal and Clinical Considerations in the Treatment of Life-Endangering Patients* (3rd ed.). Sarasota, FL: Professional Resource Press.

VandeCreek, L., Knapp, S., & Herzog, C. (1987). Malpractice risks in the treatment of dangerous patients. *Psychotherapy, 24,* 145-153.

VandenBos, G., & Duthie, R. (1986). Confronting and supporting colleagues in distress. In R. Kilburg, P. Nathan, & R. Thoreson (Eds.), *Professionals in Distress: Issues, Syndromes, and Solutions in Psychology* (pp. 211-232). Washington, DC: American Psychological Association.

Webster, N. (1956). *Webster's New Twentieth Century Dictionary* (2nd ed.). New York: World Publishing Co.

Weissman, M. L. (1991). Child custody evaluations: Fair and unfair professional practices. *Behavioral Sciences and the Law, 9*(4), 469-476.

Weithorn, L. A. (1983). Involving children in decisions affecting their own welfare. In G. Melton, G. Koocher, & M. Saks (Eds.), *Children's Competence to Consent* (pp. 235-260). New York: Plenum.

Werth, J. L., Jr., Wright, K. S., Archambault, R. J., & Bardash, R. (2003, July). When does the "duty to protect" apply with a client who has anorexia nervosa? *Counseling Psychologist, 31*(4), 427-450.

White, V. E., McCormick, L. J., & Kelly, B. L. (2003, April). Counseling clients who self-injure: Ethical considerations. *Counseling and Values, 47*(3), 220-229.

Wickline v. State of California, 228 Cal. 661 (Cal. Ct. App. 1986).

Wiens, A. (1983). Toward a conceptualization of competency assurance. *Professional Practice of Psychology, 4*(2), 1-15.

Wright, R. (1981). Psychologists and professional liability (malpractice) insurance: A retrospective review. *American Psychologist, 36,* 1485-1493.

INDEX

If You Found This Book Useful . . .

You might want to know more about our other titles.

If you would like to receive our latest catalog, please return this form:

Name: _____

Address: _____

Address: _____

City/State/Zip: _____

Telephone: (_____)_____

E-mail: _____

Fax: (_____) _____

I am a:

☐ Psychologist   ☐ Mental Health Counselor
☐ Psychiatrist   ☐ Marriage and Family Therapist
☐ School Psychologist   ☐ Not in Mental Health Field
☐ Clinical Social Worker   ☐ Other: _____

◆   ◆   ◆

Professional Resource Press
P.O. Box 15560
Sarasota, FL 34277-1560

Telephone: 800-443-3364
FAX: 941-343-9201
E-mail: orders@prpress.com
Website: http://www.prpress.com

Add A Colleague To Our Mailing List . . .

If you would like us to send our latest catalog to one of your colleagues, please return this form:

Name: _____

Address: _____

Address: _____

City/State/Zip: _____

Telephone: (_____)_____

E-mail: _____

Fax: (_____) _____

This person is a:

☐ Psychologist   ☐ Mental Health Counselor
☐ Psychiatrist   ☐ Marriage and Family Therapist
☐ School Psychologist   ☐ Not in Mental Health Field
☐ Clinical Social Worker   ☐ Other: _____

Name of person completing this form: _____

◆   ◆   ◆

Professional Resource Press
P.O. Box 15560
Sarasota, FL 34277-1560

Telephone: 800-443-3364
FAX: 941-343-9201
E-mail: orders@prpress.com
Website: http://www.prpress.com

KUGW4/01/05